Non-Invasive Respiratory Support Techniques

Non-Invasive Respiratory Support Techniques

Oxygen Therapy, Non-Invasive Ventilation and CPAP

Glenda Esmond

Respiratory Nurse Consultant
Barnet Primary Care Trust
London

and

Christine Mikelsons

Consultant Respiratory Physiotherapist
Royal Free Hampstead NHS Trust
London

(W)WILEY-BLACKWELL

A John Wiley & Sons, Ltd., Publication

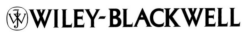

Library of Congress Cataloging-in-Publication Data

Esmond, Glenda.
  Non-invasive respiratory support techniques : oxygen therapy, non-invasive ventilation, and CPAP / Glenda Esmond and Christine Mikelsons.
       p. ; cm.
  Includes bibliographical references and index.
  ISBN 978-1-4051-3014-1 (pbk. : alk. paper) 1. Respiratory therapy. 2. Oxygen therapy. 3. Intermittent positive pressure breathing. I. Mikelsons, Christine. II. Title.
  [DNLM: 1. Respiratory Insufficiency–therapy. 2. Oxygen Inhalation Therapy–methods. 3. Positive-Pressure Respiration–methods. WF 145 E76n 2008]
  RM161.E86 2008
  615.8′36–dc22

                                                                      2008015232

A catalogue record for this book is available from the British Library.

Set in 10/13pt Palatino by Graphicraft Limited, Hong Kong
Printed in Singapore by Utopia Press Pte Ltd

1   2008

CONTENTS

CONTRIBUTORS

Glenda Esmond
Respiratory Nurse Consultant
Barnet Primary Care Trust
London

Christine Mikelsons
Consultant Respiratory Physiotherapist
Physiotherapy Department
Royal Free Hampstead NHS Trust
London

John Hurst
Senior Lecturer and Honorary Consultant Physician
Respiratory and Acute Medicine
University College London and Royal Free Hampstead NHS Trust
London

Maura McElligott
Head of Nursing
North Middlesex University Hospital NHS Trust
London

Sandra Gallacher
Practice Development Nurse
North Middlesex University Hospital NHS Trust
London

Chapter 1

CLINICAL MANAGEMENT OF RESPIRATORY FAILURE

John Hurst

This chapter provides an introduction to the clinical management of respiratory failure. Clinical management comprises both assessment and treatment, topics covered in more detail later in this book, and here the aim is to provide background knowledge on the definition of respiratory failure, and an understanding of the basic pathophysiological principles involved. The chapter concludes with some worked examples. After reading this chapter you should be able to:

- Define Type I and Type II respiratory failure.
- Understand the differences in pathogenesis between Type I and Type II respiratory failure.
- Describe the assessment and management of a patient with respiratory failure.

What is respiratory failure?

Respiratory failure may be defined as impaired pulmonary gas exchange leading to hypoxaemia (low blood oxygen tension) with or without hypercapnia (high blood carbon dioxide tension). The presence or absence of hypercapnia is used to classify respiratory failure into Type I and Type II, and this is important with regard to the likely underlying cause, and treatment, as we shall see. Type I respiratory failure is present when the partial pressure of arterial carbon dioxide ($PaCO_2$) is normal or low. Type II respiratory failure is present if the $PaCO_2$ is elevated. From this definition it will already be apparent that a key investigation in respiratory failure is blood gas analysis, both to make the diagnosis and to allow correct classification. Traditionally a partial pressure of arterial oxygen (PaO_2) <8 kPa indicates respiratory failure, but it is important to remember that PaO_2 is dependent on the fractional concentration of inspired oxygen (FiO_2) such that the 8 kPa cut-off is appropriate only for a patient breathing room air, at sea level. A normal PaO_2

under such circumstances is >12 kPa (somewhat less in older people) and the normal range for $PaCO_2$ is 4.5–6.0 kPa. We will describe in more detail later in this chapter how to identify whether a patient who is breathing supplemental oxygen has respiratory failure on the basis of blood gas analysis results.

What are the causes of respiratory failure?

The function of the respiratory system is gas exchange, but for this to be effective the individual components of the system must all be operating normally. The components are illustrated schematically in Figure 1.1, and include the conducting airways that transfer air from the outside to the gas exchanging airways, the gas-exchanging airways themselves, the respiratory muscle pump that drives air in and out of the lungs, the control system of that pump which includes the central and peripheral nervous systems, together with the pulmonary vasculature. Impairment of any one or a combination of these components might result in respiratory failure and, indeed, this provides one useful method of classifying the causes of respiratory failure as outlined in Table 1.1. One must accept, however, that this is an over-simplification and many disease processes may result in respiratory failure through a combination of mechanisms. Chronic obstructive pulmonary disease (COPD), for example, is associated with bronchoconstriction of the conducting airways, emphysema destroying the gas-exchange surface, a skeletal myopathy affecting the respiratory muscle pump and pulmonary hypertension.

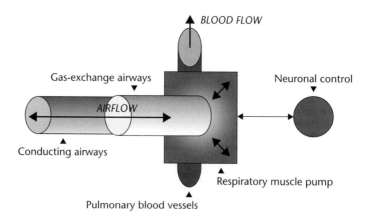

Figure 1.1 Components of the respiratory system.

Table 1.1   Causes of respiratory failure, classified by the predominant site of pathology in the respiratory system.

Conducting airways	Gas-exchange airways	Respiratory muscle pump	Neuronal control	Pulmonary blood vessels
Sleep apnoea	Pneumonia	Myopathy	Drugs	Pulmonary embolus
Upper airway obstruction	Acute respiratory distress syndrome (ARDS)	Chest wall disorders	Stroke	Pulmonary hypertension
Chronic obstructive pulmonary disease (COPD)	Pulmonary fibrosis	Neuromuscular disease	Trauma	
Asthma	Cardiac failure		Motor neurone disease Guillain–Barré syndrome	

The pathophysiology of respiratory failure

Figure 1.1 illustrates that for effective gas exchange oxygen must be transferred via the conducting airways to the gas-exchange portion of the lung, under the power of the respiratory muscle pump, which is itself controlled by the central nervous system, and into a functioning blood supply. Hypoxaemia may develop if any one or a combination of these components is damaged. In essence, there is therefore a disorder between the ventilation (gas delivery) and perfusion (blood delivery) in the lung. This is referred to as V/Q mismatch and implies that some gas-exchanging portions of the lung receive blood supply but no oxygen, and others receive oxygen and no blood supply. This explains why patients with pneumonia, for example, may be more breathless than those who have had pneumonectomy (lung removal). The pneumonectomy patient has no V/Q mismatch, whereas in pneumonia, for example, the consolidated and under-ventilated portion of the lung continues to receive blood supply, and indeed may receive more than usual as a result of the inflammatory reaction. In summary, Type I respiratory failure is usually the result of V/Q mismatch.

The situation for Type II respiratory failure is a little more complex. Carbon dioxide transfers much more easily across the alveolar–capillary barrier and excess carbon dioxide in the blood tends to represent alveolar under (hypo)ventilation. This may occur in the presence of respiratory disease but, unlike Type I respiratory failure, may also occur in lungs that are completely normal and where respiratory failure results from failure of the respiratory muscle pump. When the pump itself is normal, but is subjected to excessive demands, Type II failure may also result and our patient with pneumonia and Type I failure may progress to Type II failure if treatment is not delivered effectively.

The management of respiratory failure

The management of respiratory failure comprises two main principles: treatment aimed at any specific underlying reversible cause, and interventions aimed at supporting respiratory function to give other therapies sufficient time to be effective (or when no specific underlying cause is identifiable).

Treatment of the underlying diseases leading to respiratory failure is beyond the scope of this chapter but include, for example, antibiotics in our patient with bacterial pneumonia, and steroids with nebulised bronchodilators in exacerbations of asthma and COPD. The supportive treatments available include oxygen, and respiratory support with continuous positive airway pressure (CPAP), non-invasive ventilation (NIV) or invasive ventilation. These will be discussed in more detail later in the book, and for now we will concern ourselves with the assessment of a patient known or thought to be in respiratory failure.

Assessment of a patient with respiratory failure

Assessment comprises a clinical history (story from the patient and others, supplemented with information derived from direct questions), examination of the patient, and diagnostic investigations. The aim is to confirm the presence of respiratory failure, assess the severity, and establish an underlying diagnosis such that specific treatment can be given.

History

The principal symptoms of respiratory disease are breathlessness, cough, sputum production, wheeze and chest pain. We may add to these, those symptoms commonly associated with hypercapnia such as tiredness, morning headaches, ankle swelling, poor sleep quality and snoring.

When assessing breathlessness, a key feature is the speed of onset. The causes of respiratory failure listed in Table 1.1 vary considerably

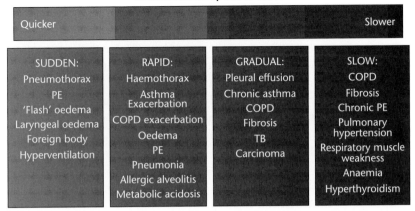

Figure 1.2   The speed of onset of breathlessness informs the likely underlying cause. PE, pulmonary embolism; COPD, chronic obstructive pulmonary disease; TB, tuberculosis.

in their speed of onset, and a schema for the onset of breathlessness is illustrated in Figure 1.2.

At the quickest, pneumothorax can occur over seconds. In contrast, the breathlessness associated with pulmonary hypertension, for example, may progress slowly over years.

In addition, one can consider the following aspects of the patient's breathlessness:

- Are the symptoms constant or variable? Variation in symptoms is typical of diseases such as asthma where the obstruction to airflow is variable. In COPD, by contrast, much of the airflow limitation is fixed and therefore symptoms are typically more constant from day to day. In addition, it is important to assess whether the symptoms are worse after a period at work, and better when on holiday, suggesting a workplace exposure.
- Are the symptoms relieved or made worse by anything the patient does. For example, weakness of the respiratory muscles may be more noticeable when the patient is lying down, 'orthopnoea'. Orthopnoea is also a feature of breathlessness in advanced heart failure.
- Is there or have there been any exposures to agents that are known to cause respiratory disease, in particular tobacco smoke, but including many others such as agents associated with asthma in the home and at work (for example animal dander), while environmental exposure to other agents such as asbestos can result in fibrosing (scarring) lung diseases.
- What are the associated symptoms? Cough and sputum, for example, may suggest COPD. Snoring may suggest sleep apnoea.

Finally, it should be emphasised that while the focus is on the cardiorespiratory system, a complete history should be obtained, and corroborated where necessary with information from others. There are many unusual causes of breathlessness and respiratory failure for which clues may be obtained in the history. One might consider, for example, information on pets at home informing on a diagnosis such as extrinsic allergic alveolitis, or a history of prior use of appetite suppressants resulting in pulmonary hypertension. Readers should refer to a standard text for further detail on the art of history taking (Douglas et al., 2005).

Examination

A complete examination should be performed, with an emphasis on the cardiorespiratory system. Again, the reader is referred to standard works which outline the principles of complete examination (Douglas et al., 2005).

Initially, the pattern, depth and rate of respiration can be observed. Likewise, the patient's body habitus (general shape and size) can be examined prior to formal calculation of the body mass index (BMI, the weight in kg divided by the square of the height in m).

Peripheral signs of respiratory disease include tar staining of the fingers, digital clubbing (typically associated with lung fibrosis, lung cancer and chronic pulmonary infections such as bronchiectasis) and the coarse flapping tremor and bounding pulse of carbon dioxide retention (Type II respiratory failure).

In the head and neck it is important to assess for clinical signs of anaemia (conjunctival pallor), central cyanosis (a much better assessment than peripheral cyanosis in the assessment of respiratory failure), elevation of the jugular venous pressure, and the shape and size of the neck. Neuromuscular diseases are important causes of respiratory failure and therefore it is important to examine for evidence of muscle wasting and fasciculation. Similarly, sleep apnoea and obesity hypoventilation syndromes can present with respiratory failure, and in addition to a general impression of BMI and neck circumference, it is important to note features such as mouth breathing, and abnormalities of the pharynx such as tonsillar enlargement.

Examination of the chest includes inspection, palpation, percussion and auscultation. The chest is inspected for scars and deformities. Palpation is used to assess the position of the mediastinum (trachea and apex beat) and to assess the depth of respiration. Percussion and auscultation are used to localise and classify the site of lung disease. The key question to ask when percussing is 'Is this resonant or is this dull', each time the chest is percussed, in comparison with the note in adjacent areas on that side of the chest, and on the contralateral side. The identification of hyper-resonant from resonant, and stony dull from dull is difficult. Similarly, when auscultating the key questions are 'Are these breath sounds normal (vesicular), normal but reduced in volume, or different'. In addition, ask 'Are there any added sounds?' such as musical wheeze, or non-musical crackles and pleural rubs. Wheeze may be diffuse or localised, and monophonic (single note) or polyphonic (multiple notes). Disease such as asthma and COPD which cause widespread narrowing of many airways produce diffuse, polyphonic wheeze. Localised, monophonic wheeze suggests localised airflow obstruction. Bronchial breathing is quite different from normal vesicular sounds and has been characterised as occurring when inspiration and expiration are of equal volume and length, when there is a pause between inspiration and expiration, and when the sounds are 'blowing' in nature.

The clinical signs may then be put together and matched to various patterns of disease, as summarised in Table 1.2. These are stereotyped, and simplified, in the table, but serve to illustrate typical patterns of disease.

Table 1.2 Stereotypical patterns of diseases in respiratory failure.

	Palpation (position of mediastinum)	**Percussion**	**Auscultation**
Normal	Not displaced	Resonant	Vesicular sounds, nil added
Large effusion	Displaced to the other side	('Stony') dull	Diminished vesicular, nil added
Pneumothorax	Displaced to the other side	('Hyper') resonant	Diminished vesicular, nil added
Collapse	Displaced to the same side	Dull	Diminished vesicular, nil added
Pneumonia	Not displaced	Dull	Bronchial sounds, with crackles
Asthma and chronic obstructive pulmonary disease	Not displaced	Resonant	Vesicular sounds, with wheeze
Heart failure	Apex displaced	Resonant	Vesicular sounds, with crackles
Fibrosis	Not displaced	Resonant	Vesicular sounds, with crackles
Pulmonary embolism	Not displaced	Resonant	Vesicular sounds, nil added ?pleural rub

Diagnostic investigations

Standard investigations in the assessment of a patient with suspected respiratory failure includes the points discussed below.

Blood gas analysis

Blood gas analysis is performed to confirm the presence of respiratory failure, inform on the likely timescale of development, and differentiate Type I from Type II disease. Pulse oximetry, which estimates oxygen saturation but gives no information on carbon dioxide, in addition to having limitations in many situations including reduced cardiac output, is often used as a screening tool. Blood gas analysis may be performed on capillary or arterial samples as described later in this book. One simplified approach to blood gas analysis is given below, and summarised in Figure 1.3.

1. Is the patient acidotic or alkalotic, or is the pH normal? An abnormal pH suggests either that the problem is new, or that a longer standing problem has become decompensated. In either event, an abnormal pH generally indicates a greater urgency for treatment.
2. When the pH is abnormal, if the direction of change of the carbon dioxide explains the abnormality seen in pH then this is a primary respiratory problem. For example, a low pH and a high carbon dioxide indicate primary respiratory acidosis.
3. Conversely, when the pH is abnormal and the direction of change is not explained by the carbon dioxide, but is explained by the direction of change in bicarbonate, then this is a primary metabolic problem. This would occur, for example, when a low pH is accompanied by a reduced bicarbonate concentration, indicating metabolic acidosis.
4. Is there a partial compensatory change in the other parameter (bicarbonate if pH explained by carbon dioxide, carbon dioxide if the pH explained by bicarbonate)?
5. If the pH is normal, is this a fully compensated acid–base disturbance manifested by abnormalities of both carbon dioxide and bicarbonate?
6. Finally, ask what is the PaO_2 and how does this relate to the FiO_2? It is possible to assess the presence of respiratory failure when patients are breathing oxygen, by calculating the A-a gradient.

$$\text{A-a gradient} = PAO_2 - (PaO_2 + PaCO_2/0.8)$$

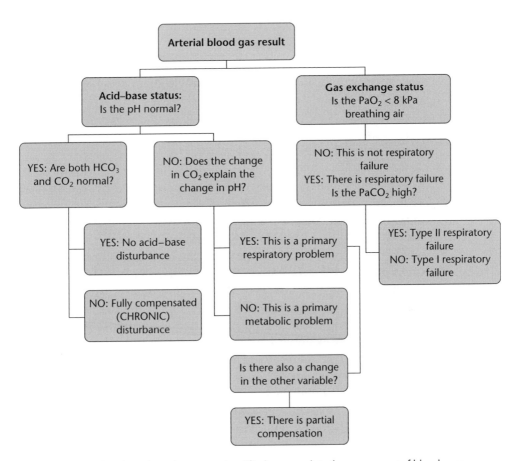

Figure 1.3 Flow chart showing a simplified approach to the assessment of blood gases.

PAO_2, or the alveolar PO_2, is calculated by expressing the FiO_2 as a percentage of 100 kPa (atmospheric pressure) – 7 kPa water vapour pressure. The normal A-a gradient is less than 3 kPa. Thus, for example, a patient who has a PaO_2 of 15 kPa and $PaCO_2$ of 4 kPa when breathing 60% oxygen has an A-a gradient of:

$$(60/100 \times (100 - 7)) - (15 + 4/0.8) = 55.8 - 20 = 35.8 \text{ kPa}$$

This is abnormal and therefore indicates the presence of respiratory failure. A simplified approach, used in the definition of acute lung injury and the acute respiratory distress syndrome, is to calculate the PaO_2/FiO_2 ratio. The definition of acute lung injury includes PaO_2/FiO_2 < 27 kPa (200 mmHg).

Full blood count

Anaemia is a cause of breathlessness, and respiratory failure can be associated with the development of polycythaemia which may require specific treatment.

Lung function tests

Spirometry (forced expiratory volume in one second (FEV_1) and forced vital capacity (FVC)) will differentiate obstructive from restrictive diseases, a crucial distinction in respiratory medicine that is discussed further below. Static lung volumes such as total lung capacity give additional information on conditions associated with scarring and gas trapping. Assessing the carbon monoxide transfer factor (a proxy for the ability of oxygen to cross the alveolar–capillary barrier) can aid differentiation of restrictive defects due to lung diseases (such as pulmonary fibrosis, where the barrier is thickened) from extra-thoracic restriction in, for example, neuromuscular disease where the problem is one of mismatched demand and ability of the respiratory muscle pump to achieve adequate gas exchange.

The distinction between obstructive and restrictive patterns on spirometry is important in establishing a differential diagnosis. These are best considered by reference to a flow-volume loop, which will be provided by many spirometry services. A hypothetical normal flow volume loop, and those that may be obtained in obstructive and restrictive diseases are illustrated in Figure 1.4. Note that flow is plotted on the y-axis, and a positive flow indicates expiration, a negative flow is inspiration. The x-axis represents lung volume, with total lung capacity at the origin, and distance travelled along the x-axis indicating the vital capacity (VC, total amount of air that can be moved in and out of the lung). The total lung capacity is made up of VC and residual volume, the volume of air that remains in the chest after a maximal expiration. In the normal loop (a), starting from a maximal inspiration where the axes cross, the maximum (peak) expiratory flow rate is achieved rapidly, before it tails off more gradually to the end of expiration. This expiratory limb, above the axis, is roughly triangular in shape. The inspiratory limb is below the x-axis. It takes longer to reach the maximal inspiratory flow, which is lower in magnitude than the maximal expiratory flow, and the shape of this curve is roughly semi-circular.

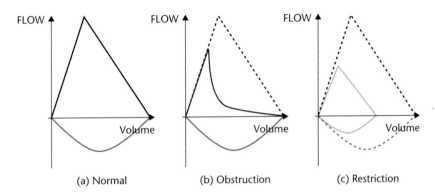

Figure 1.4   Stereotyped flow-volume loops in a normal subject (a), subject with an obstructive lung deficit (b) and subject with a restrictive lung deficit (c). See text for details.

In diseases characterised by obstruction to the flow of air (Figure 1.4b), and therefore those typically affecting the bronchial tree such as asthma and COPD, the peak expiratory flow rate is reduced and in early expiration, collapse of the airways results in a rapid reduction in expiratory flow rate and a characteristic 'scalloped' shape to the curve. Note that vital capacity, the distance on the y-axis, is not reduced and therefore expressing FEV_1/FVC in an obstructive condition results in a lower than normal value. In restrictive lung diseases, the total lung capacity has been affected and is reduced considerably as shown in Figure 1.4c where the distance on the y-axis is reduced. Compare the patient's trace to the normal trace shown in dotted lines. However, the relative flow rates throughout inspiration and expiration are not altered, and the shape of the trace is a miniaturised version of the normal trace. Expressing FEV_1/FVC here, in a restrictive condition, will result in a normal ratio as both FEV_1 and FVC have been reduced. Restrictive conditions can be caused by lung pathology such as the fibrotic lung diseases, but a restrictive pattern may also result when the respiratory muscle pump is unable to meet the demands placed on it, for example in the case of respiratory muscle weakness, or gross obesity. Fortunately it is possible to distinguish lung ('thoracic') from other ('extra-thoracic') restriction, by reference to the measurement of gas transfer, as described above. Readers requiring further detail are referred to a standard work on pulmonary function testing (Ruppel, 2003).

A simplified strategy for the interpretation of lung function tests might therefore be as follows, assuming that the test is of an acceptable technical quality.

1.   Examine the FEV_1 and FVC, expressed as a percentage of predicted for that patient's age, sex, height and race; <80% predicted is considered abnormal.
2.   If the FEV_1 or FVC are abnormal, examine the FEV_1/FVC ratio. For reasons described above, in relation to the flow volume loop, a ratio >0.7 implies a restrictive disease (either thoracic or extra-thoracic), while a ratio <0.7 implies an obstructive disease. The ratio is not generally helpful if both FEV_1 and FVC are normal (>80%).
3.   If there is evidence of airflow obstruction, consider whether there is additional supporting evidence such as the shape of the flow-volume loop, which can be reflected mathematically by examining the flow-rate at between 25% and 75% of VC, the FEF25–75, which would be significantly reduced.
4.   In airflow obstruction, a bronchodilator reversibility test is sometimes performed in which spirometry is repeated before and after administration of a bronchodilator such as salbutamol. Classically, COPD is characterised by fixed airflow obstruction, and asthma by reversible airflow obstruction, although these concepts are currently being challenged (Calverley et al., 2003). The cut-off for reversibility is also controversial but might typically be around 200 ml or 15% change in absolute FEV_1.
5.   If there is evidence of restriction, consider whether there is additional supporting evidence such as reduced total lung capacity.
6.   In a restrictive disease, examining the gas transfer can differentiate between thoracic and extra-thoracic restriction.

Chest X-ray

Chest X-rays are performed to assess the appearance of the underlying lungs. One simplified strategy for interpretation of a chest X-ray is given below.

1.   Check that this is the correct X-ray film (name and date).
2.   Assess if the film is technically adequate (that is, exclude rotation by looking at the ends of the clavicles in relation to the vertebral spinous processes, ensure there is adequate penetration such that the vertebral bodies are just visible behind the heart, ensure there has been an adequate inspiration and that all the lung fields have been included on the film). A film that is generally too white is described as under-penetrated (the X-ray dose was too low) and a film that is too black is over-penetrated (the X-ray dose was too high).

3. Assess whether the film has been taken in the antero-posterior (AP) or postero-anterior (PA) direction (which is important, for example, on the ability to comment on heart size) and whether the X-ray was taken with the patient erect or supine.
4. Systematically examine the lung fields, soft tissues and bones for abnormalities. In general, the lungs should be of approximately equal density from top to bottom and left to right.
5. Describe the shape, size, density, location and distribution of any abnormalities.
6. Check whether there are any old X-ray films available for comparison.

Specialist investigations

The investigations described above will be important in most patients presenting with respiratory failure. Many patients, as we shall see in the worked examples below, require more specialised tests, the detailed description of which is outwith the scope of this chapter. However, these may include:

- Further **lung imaging** – for example with a high-resolution chest computed tomography (CT) scan of the chest.
- More complex **lung function assessment** – for example testing the strength of respiratory muscles, with mouth (inspiratory) pressure.
- **Sleep study** to investigate the possibility of diagnoses such as the obstructive sleep apnoea syndrome (OSAS).
- **Trans-thoracic echocardiography** to inform on cardiac function, perhaps progressing in selected patients to further tests such as serum brain natriuretic protein (BNP) assay (which is elevated in heart failure), or cardiac catheterisation and assessment of pulmonary artery pressure.

Summary

Respiratory failure may be defined as impaired pulmonary gas exchange leading to hypoxaemia with or without hypercapnia. Type I respiratory failure is present when the partial pressure of arterial carbon dioxide ($PaCO_2$) is normal or low. Type II respiratory failure is present if the $PaCO_2$ is elevated. Impairment of any one or a combination of the conducting airways, the gas-exchanging airways, the respiratory muscle pump and the control system of that pump, together with the pulmonary vasculature may result in respiratory failure. The assessment of a patient with suspected respiratory failure includes the history, examination, and diagnostic investigations. The aim is to confirm the presence of respiratory failure, assess the severity, and establish an underlying diagnosis such that specific treatment can be given. The management of respiratory failure comprises two main principles: treatment aimed at any specific underlying reversible cause, and interventions aimed at supporting respiratory function to give other therapies sufficient time to be effective or when no such specific cause has been identified. Such principles of investigation and management are discussed in more detail in the subsequent chapters.

This chapter concludes with some worked examples of patients with respiratory failure, illustrating how the principles of assessment described above may be applied in clinical practice.

Case studies

Case study 1.1

A 63-year-old woman makes an appointment to see you, her primary care provider, as she has noticed increasing breathlessness when out shopping over the past few months.

What are the important points you will wish to address in the history?

The key to assessing breathlessness is to establish the speed of onset, and any associated symptoms. Here the onset is over months, which changes the likely diagnosis in comparison with breathlessness that has occurred over a few hours. On direct questioning, she also has a daily cough productive of white sputum, and wheeze but no chest pain. She does not complain of ankle swelling, or morning headaches. She is a little tired but says that her sleep quality is good. She does not think that she snores. The breathlessness is not variable, or worse in any particular position. She can lie flat without breathlessness. She started smoking aged 14, up to 20 cigarettes per day, and stopped at age 54. She had hay fever as a child. There do not seem to be any current environmental factors affecting her disease.

What do you think the most likely cause of her breathlessness is, and how will you establish this?

The slow progression of symptoms that do not vary, and a supporting significant exposure to tobacco smoke, make COPD the most likely diagnosis. Smoking exposure can be quantified by calculating the 'pack-years' smoked. This is calculated by dividing the number of cigarettes smoked per day by 20, and multiplying this by the number of years smoked. To develop COPD, it would be unusual to have less than 20 pack-years exposure and this woman has 40 pack-years. The hay fever as a child does raise the possibility that this may be asthma, as asthma is associated with other atopic diseases including hay fever. Although clinical examination is important and the finding of wheeze on examination may help, the diagnosis of COPD can only be confirmed by performing spirometry. The differentiation from asthma can be challenging and may require a formal reversibility test in response to nebulised bronchodilators or steroids, or daily peak-flow monitoring to assess for any day-to-day variation in symptoms.

You have spirometry available in the surgery and her results are as follows: FEV_1 0.63 l or 33% predicted, FVC 2.01 l or 87% predicted, and FEV_1/FVC ratio 0.31. Interpret these results.

Assuming the spirometry is technically adequate, the FEV_1 is low and FVC is normal (>80%), with a FEV_1/FVC ratio <0.7 suggesting an obstructive process. If a flow volume loop was available it may show the characteristic 'scallop' shape. After nebulised salbutamol, her FEV_1 increased to 0.66 l but as this is <200 ml and 15%, the disease is not considered 'reversible' and COPD is the most likely diagnosis. Criteria, and indeed the concept of reversibility remains a subject of debate.

What other tests are indicated?

The degree of impairment of FEV_1 is used to classify the severity of COPD in current international guidelines (National Institute for Clinical Excellence, 2004; Global Initiative for Chronic Obstructive Lung Disease, 2007). With an FEV_1 of 33%, this woman has severe COPD and it would be appropriate to perform oxygen saturations (to exclude respiratory failure), a full blood count (to exclude anaemia) and a chest X-ray (to exclude other complicating diagnoses, and which may show features compatible with COPD). Her haemoglobin concentration was normal, and her chest X-ray is shown in Figure 1.5.

Interpret the X-ray.

Figure 1.5 is a PA erect film of reasonable technical quality. The lungs are hyper-expanded in keeping with a diagnosis of COPD, there are no focal lung lesions, and the bones and soft tissues appear normal.

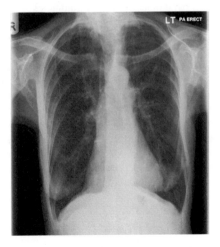

Figure 1.5 Chest X-ray, Case 1.1.

Case study 1.1   (Continued)

Her oxygen saturation breathing room air was 92%. What would you do next?

An oxygen saturation of 92% equates, approximately, to an arterial oxygen tension of 8 kPa. The patient may therefore have respiratory failure, but this needs to be confirmed with blood gas analysis, which will also inform on the carbon dioxide levels and allow differentiation of Type I respiratory failure from Type II respiratory failure.

She was referred to her local oxygen assessment service and the following blood gas results were returned. What is your interpretation of these?

pH	7.368
PaO_2 (11–15 kPa)	7.71 kPa
$PaCO_2$ (4.5–6.0 kPa)	8.0 kPa
HCO_3^- (24–30 mmol/l)	32.3 mmol/l
FiO_2	0.21

The pH is normal so by definition she is neither acidotic nor alkalotic, however both the HCO_3^- and $PaCO_2$ are abnormal in keeping with a fully compensated and therefore chronic acid–base disturbance. It is not possible, theoretically, to say whether this is a primary respiratory acidosis with complete metabolic compensation, or a primary metabolic alkalosis with complete respiratory compensation. However, the latter does not occur, so this is indeed a fully compensated respiratory acidosis. The PaO_2 is <8 kPa breathing room air, so she has respiratory failure, and the $PaCO_2$ is elevated defining this as Type II respir-atory failure.

What are the principles of management?

Recall that the management of respiratory failure comprises two main principles: treatment aimed at any specific underlying reversible cause, and interventions aimed at supporting respiratory function. Therefore, her COPD therapy should be optimised by a specialist in this condition. If, after this, she remains hypoxic then current guidelines support the use of domiciliary oxygen therapy for patients with COPD who have a PaO_2 < 7.3 kPa breathing room air, twice, when clinically stable. This criteria is raised to <8 kPa where there is clinical evidence of right heart failure. Oxygen is titrated to correct the PaO_2 to >8 kPa and evidence suggests that it should be used for at least 15 hours in every 24-hour period (Nocturnal Oxygen Therapy Trial Group, 1980; Medical Research Council Working Party, 1981). If she is active, she may also benefit from a portable (ambulatory) supply. Assessments will need to be performed to ensure that increasing her FiO_2 does not result in a rise in $PaCO_2$ of >1 kPa or fall in pH (decompensation). Acutely, for example at an exacerbation, an inability to achieve adequate oxygenation without a rise in $PaCO_2$ and fall in pH would be an indication for non-invasive ventilation. The benefits of domiciliary non-invasive ventilation for newly diagnosed chronic Type II respiratory failure in COPD are less clear and this subject remains controversial.

Case study 1.2

As a member of staff working in emergency medicine, you are asked to see a 24-year-old man who has walked into the emergency department, complaining of breathlessness, a cough productive of green sputum, right-sided pleuritic chest pains and fever.

What are the important points you will wish to address in the history?

Again, the key to assessing breathlessness is to establish the speed of onset, and any associated symptoms. In this case the onset is much more acute, over a few days, and he is previously fit and active, with a physical job as a builder. The cough, phlegm and fever suggest infection of the airways (bronchitis) or lung parenchyma (pneumonia) but the chest pain suggests the latter as there is peripheral, pleural irritation and this is localising to the right side. 'Pleuritic' pain is typically worse on inspiration and may 'catch' the patient if they are asked to take a deep breath in. As always, it is important to be thorough and, for example, his job as a builder may result in exposure to various occupational dusts that could cause diseases of the lung.

On examination, his temperature is 38.3°C, his heart rate is 100/minute, and his blood pressure is 100/60 mmHg. His respiratory rate is 20/minute and his oxygen saturation is 94% breathing room air. Interpret these vital signs, and outline your immediate plan.

These signs are consistent with a diagnosis of pneumonia: the patient is pyrexial, tachycardic, has borderline hypotension, tachypnoea and hypoxia. He needs a rapid but complete physical assessment, and urgent investigations and treatment. Oxygen therapy should be given to maintain a target saturation of around 95%, and in the absence of signs of heart failure it would be sensible to commence intravenous fluids to support his cardiovascular system, aiming to see a reduction in heart rate and increase in blood pressure.

On examination of the chest, expansion is greater on the left than the right, the mediastinum is not displaced, the left side is more resonant than the right, and while breath sounds on the left are normal those on the right sound blowing and there are coarse crackles present. Interpret the clinical findings.

These findings are consistent with right sided consolidation and a diagnosis of pneumonia. In pneumonia the lung parenchyma fills with an inflammatory reaction (becomes 'consolidated') and this accounts for the reduction in expansion on that side because not as much air is moving in and out. However, there is no mediastinal shift as there is no overall change in volume of the lung. The reduction in percussion note, termed 'dull', is because the underlying lung is now airless, and the 'blowing' breath sounds are typical of 'bronchial breathing' where the consolidated lung is transmitting the sounds of airflow in the larger airways to the surface of the lung. Bronchial breathing is also characterised by an audible pause between inspiration and expiration (this does not normally occur), and inspiration and expiration being of equal length (normally expiration is longer). Bronchial breathing is characteristic of pneumonia, and coarse crackles are also often heard.

Case study 1.2   (Continued)

What investigations would you perform to confirm this, and to assess the severity of the disease process?

This patient should have a full blood count, urea and electrolyte assay, liver function tests, C-reactive protein and blood cultures. An arterial blood gas should be performed. He should have a chest X-ray and an electrocardiogram (ECG). Urine should be collected for urinalysis and detection of pneumococcal and legionella antigens. Sputum should be sent for microscopy, culture and sensitivity. The aim of these tests is to confirm the clinical suspicion of pneumonia, to attempt to identify the causative organism, and to assess the severity of the disease. National and international guidelines for the treatment of pneumonia also exist (British Thoracic Society, 2004; Infectious Disease Society of America, 2007) and these include severity scales. The simplest to use is the CURB-65 (Lim et al., 2003):

Score one point for each of the following:

CONFUSION (abbreviated mental test score <8)
UREA >7 mmol/l
RESPIRATORY RATE >30/min
BLOOD PRESSURE <90 systolic and/or <60 diastolic
>65 years old.

Mortality is related to the score such that

Score 0	0.7%
Score 1	3.2%
Score 2	13.0%
Score 3	17.0%
Score 4	41.5%
Score 5	57.0%

In this example, a points is scored for Blood Pressure but not Confusion, Urea (if normal), Respiratory Rate or Age and the total score is therefore 1 representing a low risk of death.

Interpret the chest X-ray.

Figure 1.6 is an erect PA chest X-ray that is adequately penetrated and not rotated, but it is not perfect as it is not possible to see the lung apices. There are ECG electrodes visible in an arc around the left chest wall, and a left-sided nipple ring. The most obvious area of abnormality is an area of dense, confluent shadowing in the right lower zone. This has a horizontal upper border (representing the horizontal fissure). The right heart border is obscured suggesting that the process is anterior and in contact with the heart border, and there are air bronchograms visible. This is the appearance of a right middle lobe pneumonia. Air bronchograms are also typical of pneumonia. They appear as branching black lines within the consolidated white lung, and represent patent larger airways entering an area of alveoli that are consolidated.

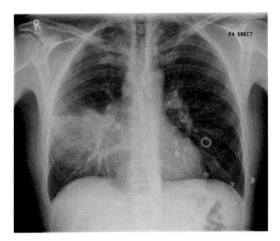

Figure 1.6   Chest X-ray, Case 1.2.

Arterial blood gas analysis is given below. Interpret the blood gas results. Why is he breathless?

pH	7.40
PaO_2 (11–15 kPa)	8.2 kPa
$PaCO_2$ (4.5–6.0 kPa)	3.8 kPa
HCO_3^- (24–30 mmol/l)	22.0 mmol/l
FiO_2	0.50

The pH is normal so by definition he is neither acidotic nor alkalotic, but both the HCO_3^- and $PaCO_2$ are abnormal suggesting a fully compensated acid–base disturbance. This could be a primary respiratory alkalosis with metabolic compensation, or a primary metabolic acidosis with respiratory compensation. Either can occur in pneumonia, as systemic infection can result in a metabolic (lactic) acidosis, and respiratory alkalosis may be seen if ventilatory drive is increased in an attempt to maintain blood oxygen tensions. The PaO_2 is >8 kPa but the patient is breathing supplemental oxygen, so an assessment of respiratory failure will need to consider the A-a gradient. This is calculated using the formula given below:

A-a gradient $= PAO_2 - (PaO_2 + PaCO_2/0.8)$

and PAO_2, or the alveolar PO_2, is calculated by expressing the FiO_2 as a % of 100 kPa (atmospheric pressure) – 7 kPa water vapour pressure. Therefore:

A-a $= (50/100 (100 - 7)) - (8.2 + (3.8/0.8)) = 33.55$ kPa

The A-a gradient here is 33.55 kPa, and therefore elevated. The $PaCO_2$ is low defining this as Type I respiratory failure. The patient is breathless because his right middle lobe is full of pus, however this alone is an insufficient explanation as patients can tolerate lobectomy very well. A better explanation would be V/Q mismatch, such that the affected part of the lung, not taking part in gas exchange, is preferentially receiving the blood supply as a result of inflammatory vasodilation.

Case study 1.2 (Continued)

How should he be managed?

Once again, the management principles are to treat the underlying cause and to support respiratory function until clinical improvement. The patient will require intravenous antibiotics for the right middle lobe pneumonia, and intravenous fluids to support his cardiovascular system. Regarding the respiratory failure, he is at present maintaining his $PaO_2 > 8$ kPa and therefore it would be appropriate to continue the 50% oxygen. An alternative would be to apply continuous positive airway pressure (CPAP) which is an effective treatment for Type I respiratory failure and may allow reduction in FiO_2 and increase in PaO_2.

Case study 1.3

A 74-year-old man is referred by his GP to the respiratory outpatient department for assessment of breathlessness. He has been getting progressively breathless for years, and it is now occurring on minimal exertion. It also occurs when lying down, and he has occasionally woken up from sleep feeling breathless, with the production of pink, frothy sputum. At other times he has a cough productive of some green phlegm, but this has not changed recently. He does not have any chest pain or wheeze. He has a past medical history of atrial fibrillation, ischaemic heart disease (including a non-ST elevation myocardial infarction 3 years ago) and late-onset diabetes mellitus. He stopped smoking 10 years ago but smoked 30 cigarettes per day for 40 years. He is a retired mechanic. On direct questioning he has gained 2 kg in weight over the past week and snores loudly.

Interpret the history.

This case is complex, and it is likely that his breathlessness is multi-factorial. The history of ischaemic heart disease, orthopnoea, paroxysmal nocturnal dyspnoea and weight gain suggest decompensated cardiac failure. However, with a significant smoking history (60 pack-years) and chronic sputum production he may also have COPD. His previous occupation as a mechanic may have resulted in exposure to asbestos. In addition, a history of snoring could suggest OSAS.

On examination, he was obese (BMI 30 kg/m²) and breathless at rest. He was apyrexial. His heart rate was 90/minute and irregularly irregular. His blood pressure was 134/76 lying. His respiratory rate was 26/minute and his saturation was 90% breathing room air. Positive findings on examination of the cardiovascular system included a pan-systolic murmur, pitting oedema on the thigh, and bilateral expiratory polyphonic wheeze. Do the examination findings modify the differential diagnosis?

No, this is still likely to be multi-factorial. There is evidence to support diagnoses of both cardiac failure, and COPD, and in addition there is a heart valve lesion. The patient's high BMI increases the likelihood of diagnosing sleep apnoea.

What investigations should be ordered and why?

When breathlessness is likely to be multi-factorial, it is often necessary to perform a variety of tests. Initially, some simple investigations would be appropriate which might include a full blood count (to exclude anaemia), arterial blood gas analysis (as he is hypoxic on air and possibly has respiratory failure), ECG (to examine the heart rhythm), chest X-ray, lung function tests and echocardiogram (given the murmur and peripheral oedema which raise the possibility of cardiac dysfunction). Depending on the results of these it may be necessary to perform more detailed studies.

The initial investigations show that the haemoglobin in normal. The ECG confirmed atrial fibrillation with a rate of 80/minute. The echocardiogram reported an ejection fraction of 45% with mild mitral regurgitation. The arterial blood gas, lung function tests and chest X-ray are shown below. Interpret these results.

pH	7.350
PaO_2 (11–15 kPa)	6.47 kPa
$PaCO_2$ (4.5–6.0 kPa)	8.34 kPa
HCO_3^- (24–30 mmol/l)	28.9 mmol/l
FiO_2	0.21
FEV_1	1.30 l (60.3% predicted)
FVC	2.61 l (91.9% predicted)
FEV_1/FVC	49.66%
Lung volumes	Not reported
TL_{CO}	3.64 mmol/min/kPa (55.0% predicted)
K_{CO}	0.93 mmol/min/kPa/l (78.4% predicted)

The blood gas results indicate fully compensated Type II respiratory failure (normal pH but raised $PaCO_2$ and raised bicarbonate; PaO_2 < 8 kPa on air). The lung function tests demonstrate an obstructive pathology (FEV_1/FVC < 0.7 or 70%), but the correction of transfer factor also suggests a degree of extrathoracic restriction. The chest X-ray (Figure 1.7) is a PA erect film that is somewhat under-penetrated (too white) and was reported by the radiologist as showing cardiomegaly (the heart size is greater than 50% the distance across the lungs at that point), bilateral calcified pleural plaques (one is clearly visible one-third of the way down the pleural border on the left, for example) and pleural thickening consistent with the patient's asbestos exposure.

What further investigations may now assist?

This case illustrates the important points that breathlessness may sometimes be multi-factorial, requiring multiple investigations, and that investigations can sometimes give results that conflict with the clinical picture.

Regarding cardiac function, the relatively normal echocardiogram is inconsistent with the clinical findings of oedema, and the patient is known to have ischaemic heart disease. It is often technically difficult to perform echocardiography in subjects with COPD as the chest may be hyper-expanded. It would therefore be important to examine the echocardiography report for comments about the confidence of the results. In addition, given the clinical discrepancy, one may also wish to seek additional evidence of heart failure and for this reason a serum BNP (brain natriuretic peptide) assay could be requested. BNP is released by the ventricles of the heart

Case study 1.3 (Continued)

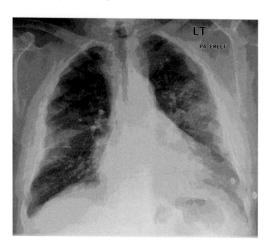

Figure 1.7 Chest X-ray, Case 1.3.

when they are stretched, as occurs in heart failure. Like all tests, however, the sensitivity and specificity are not perfect.

Regarding the lung function, a reversibility test was performed and this showed no significant response in FEV_1 and therefore these results are consistent with a degree of COPD. However, the FEV_1 is 60% predicted, suggesting that the disease is of only moderate severity and it would therefore be most unusual for COPD alone to result in hypercapnic respiratory failure without additional diagnoses being present. The history of snoring suggested sleep apnoea and a sleep study subsequently confirmed the OSAS. Finally, while the extra-thoracic restriction may just have reflected his increased BMI, the asbestos exposure and pleural thickening visible on the chest X-ray raised the possibility of more extensive pleural disease. This was investigated further with a high resolution CT scan of the chest that confirmed significant, circumferential pleural thickening.

Why was this patient breathless and how should he be treated?

The features contributing to this patient's breathlessness include raised BMI, moderate COPD, possible cardiac dysfunction, extensive pleural thickening secondary to asbestos exposure and OSAS. Management is therefore aimed at optimising all these diagnoses but the presence of Type II respiratory failure suggests the need for ventilatory support. Simple OSAS may be treated effectively with nasal CPAP but in this case where there is co-existent cardiac and respiratory disease, and Type II respiratory failure, it is preferable to establish the patient on non-invasive ventilation. Despite extensive encouragement and training this patient tolerated non-invasive ventilation poorly and the decision was made not to persist with the treatment. Application of 24% oxygen did not result in decompensation and he was eventually discharged home with long-term oxygen therapy, to use for at least 15 hours per 24-hour period, including the overnight period when desaturations are more likely.

Case study 1.4

A 32-year-old woman with a congenital kyphoscoliosis is referred to the respiratory outpatient department because of progressive breathlessness. She is 26 weeks' pregnant and, prior to the pregnancy, was not limited by dyspnoea.

Outline your initial approach to her management.

As with all these cases, the initial approach comprises a complete history and examination, followed by appropriate general and specific investigations.

On specific questioning the breathlessness had been slowly progressive from the tenth week of her pregnancy. The severity did not vary aside from this gradual progression, though it was worse on lying down and easier when standing. She had never smoked and there were no apparent occupational or environmental exposures to potential toxins. There were no associated symptoms.

On examination the kyphoscoliosis and gravid uterus were apparent. With the exception of reduced oxygen saturation while breathing room air, at 93%, examination of the cardiorespiratory system was otherwise normal. In particular, her conjunctivae were not pale and there was no peripheral oedema or signs to suggest deep vein thrombosis.

Suggest a differential diagnosis and plan of investigation.

The differential diagnosis here remains wide, and in addition to the conditions described above one must also consider conditions connected with the patient's pregnancy and kyphoscoliosis. Patients with severe kyphoscoliosis can develop respiratory failure, especially nocturnal hypoventilation, that can be remarkably asymptomatic. It is possible that her pregnant uterus is now further compromising her respiratory function. However, pregnancy can also be associated with anaemia, and an increased risk of thrombo-embolic disease, and such diagnoses must also be considered.

Appropriate initial investigations would therefore include full blood count, blood gas analysis, chest radiograph (with shielding of the fetus) and spirometry.

Blood gas analysis revealed a normal pH, PaO_2 of 10.2 kPa and $PaCO_2$ of 5.8 kPa while breathing room air. The spirometry is given below. Her haemoglobin, and chest X-ray, except for the kyphoscoliosis, were normal. Interpret the results.

FEV_1	0.77 l (34% predicted)
FVC	0.87 l (33% predicted)
FEV_1/FVC	88.51%

The normal full blood count excludes anaemia, and the normal X-ray a range of intrinsic lung diseases. Her blood gases demonstrate hypercapnia which, as the pH is normal, must be chronic. The spirometry is consistent with a restrictive process and, in the absence of evidence suggesting intrinsic lung disease the most likely explanation is indeed a worsening of kyphoscoliosis-associated respiratory impairment due to the pregnant uterus. This would also be in keeping with the history of a positional worsening of symptoms.

Case study 1.4   (Continued)

How could this be confirmed?

A sleep study would confirm nocturnal hypoventilation, which is the commonest respiratory complication of kyphoscoliosis. In this case, the sleep study did indeed confirm significant desaturations and the patient was managed successfully with non-invasive ventilation through to an elective caesarean section performed at 36 weeks' gestation. Non-invasive ventilation was continued for a further 1 week post partum. Four months later her spirometry was as below, and she had returned to her baseline functional capacity.

FEV_1	0.80 l (35% predicted)
FVC	1.00 l (38% predicted)
FEV_1/FVC	80.00%

Interpret the spirometry.

Although improved following delivery, the spirometry remains abnormal and is still consistent with a restrictive process. Assessment of gas transfer would be useful to confirm that this is indeed extra-thoracic restriction. A repeat sleep study would also be appropriate and, if nocturnal desaturations are still present, nocturnal non-invasive ventilation should be continued to prevent the long-term complication of cor pulmonale.

References

British Thoracic Society (2004) *Guidelines for the Management of Community Acquired Pneumonia in Adults*. Available at: www.brit-thoracic.org.uk/ClinicalInformation/Pneumonia/PneumoniaGuidelines/tabid/136/Default.aspx (accessed 19 May 2008).

Calverley, P.M., Burge, P.S., Spenser, S., Anderson, J.A. & Jones, P.W. (2003) Bronchodilator reversibility testing in chronic obstructive pulmonary disease. *Thorax*, **58**, 659–664.

Douglas, G., Nicol, S. & Robertson, C. (2005) *MacLeod's Clinical Examination*, 11th edn. Churchill Livingstone, Edinburgh.

Global Initiative for Chronic Obstructive Lung Disease (2007) *Global Strategy for the Diagnosis, Prevention and Management of COPD*. Available at: www.goldcopd.org

Infectious Disease Society of America (2007) American Thoracic Society Consensus Guidelines on the Management of Community-Acquired Pneumonia in Adults. *Clinical Infectious Diseases*, **44**, S27–S72.

Lim, W.S., van der Eerden, M.M., Laing, R. et al. (2003) Defining community acquired pneumonia severity on presentation to hospital: an international derivation and validation study. *Thorax*, **58**, 377–382.

Medical Research Council Working Party (1981) Long-term domiciliary oxygen therapy in chronic hypoxic cor pulmonale complicating chronic bronchitis and emphysema. *Lancet*, **i**, 681–686.

National Institute for Clinical Excellence (2004) Chronic obstructive pulmonary disease: national clinical guideline for management of chronic obstructive pulmonary disease in adults in primary and secondary care. *Thorax*, **59** (Suppl I).

Nocturnal Oxygen Therapy Trial Group (1980) Continuous or nocturnal oxygen in hypoxaemic chronic obstructive lung disease. *Annals of Internal Medicine*, **93**, 391–398.

Ruppel, G.L. (ed.) (2003) *Manual of Pulmonary Function Testing*, 8th edn. Mosby, London.

Chapter 2

ARTERIAL BLOOD GAS ANALYSIS

With contribution from Maura McElligott and
Sandra Gallacher

Arterial blood gases are an essential component of managing patients who are in respiratory failure and requiring non-invasive respiratory support, including oxygen therapy, non-invasive ventilation (NIV) and continuous positive airway pressure (CPAP). Healthcare professionals therefore require an understanding of:

- Acid–base balance
- Pulse oximetry
- Blood gas sampling techniques
- Interpretation of arterial blood gases

Acid–base physiology

In terms of clinical care, the two most important areas for concern when interpreting acid–base physiology are the:

- Chemical and physiological mechanisms that maintain a stable hydrogen ion concentration.
- Pathological processes that alter hydrogen ion concentrations during disease (Abelow, 1998).

Commonly referred to as 'acid–base disorders' or 'acid–base disturbances', changes in the acid–base balance can significantly affect the course of illness and the patient's recovery (Middleston et al., 2006).

Acid–base balance is a reflection of the hydrogen ion concentration in the body and is measured by a scale referred to as the pH. The pH is the negative logarithm of the concentration of hydrogen ions, which means that as the hydrogen ion concentration increases, the pH will decrease. Conversely, if the hydrogen ion concentration decreases then the pH will increase. The human body only operates within a very narrow pH range (pH 7.35–7.45), which is kept constant by the balance of acid and base in the body. Any deviation from this range can cause significant physiological problems (Cooper, 2004). Consequently, several different mechanisms are available to regulate pH. If one mechanism is insufficient, another can compensate. An acid is a substance that releases hydrogen ions when it dissociates in solution. A base is a substance that can accept or bind to these hydrogen ions. Acids are produced by the body as an end-product of metabolism (Cooper, 2004). This acid has to be removed or neutralised to maintain the pH constant within the acceptable pH range. The acids produced include:

- Hydrochloric acid
- Lactic acid
- Keto acids
- Uric acid
- Carbonic acid

The amount of acid produced varies, and in health the buffer systems are able to maintain acid–base balance (Watson, 2000). The respiratory and renal systems work continually as the main buffers to maintain the body within a normal acid–base balance that provides a suitable internal environment for the optimal functioning of all metabolic processes. When this balance is disrupted due to disease or illness, physiological mechanisms are triggered to restore acid–base balance. Lactic acidosis is produced when cells respire anaerobically and can indicate a state where tissues are receiving an inadequate supply of oxygen due to poor perfusion or poor oxygenation. This could be the result of hypovolaemia or hypoxia (Middleston et al., 2006). The pH is determined by the levels of carbon dioxide and bicarbonate. Carbon dioxide is eliminated through the respiratory system by adequate alveolar ventilation, hence is controlled through the lungs. By increasing respiration and ventilation, more carbon dioxide can be expelled. If needed, respiration and ventilation can then be reduced. Bicarbonate is regulated by the renal system (Abelow, 1998). Bicarbonate ions are filtered from the blood by the glomerulus, where they enter the lumen of the renal tubule. The ions are then reabsorbed across the tubule wall, thus regulating the bicarbonate level. The pH can also be regulated by buffers contained in the blood (Abelow, 1998) with the lungs and kidneys being the primary organs maintaining acid–base regulation.

An imbalance of the acid–base balance results in either acidosis (pH < 7.35) or alkalosis (pH > 7.45), and this can be a result of a respiratory or a metabolic problem.

Respiratory acidosis

Respiratory acidosis is the result of insufficient alveolar ventilation. When gaseous exchange is insufficient to excrete the metabolic products of carbon dioxide, there is rapid accumulation of this gas, leading to hypercapnia (Heuther, 1998) and respiratory acidosis (Woodrow, 2004). There are two primary causes of respiratory acidosis:

- Pulmonary
- Non-pulmonary

Pulmonary causes

Pulmonary causes of respiratory acidosis can be as a result of acute or chronic lung conditions, as outlined in Table 2.1.

Acute lung conditions usually have a rapid onset and limited duration, which is usually reversed by treatment of the underlying cause. This results in an increase in the work of breathing by causing obstruction or restriction of the air passages, or by increasing the amount of ventilation needed to allow gas exchange (Heuther, 1998). Box 2.1 lists the physiological causes of respiratory acidosis. Severe reduction of respiratory muscle function can be caused by electrolyte depletion, in particular

Table 2.1 Acute and chronic pulmonary causes of respiratory acidosis.

Acute lung conditions	Chronic lung conditions
Pneumonia	Chronic obstructive pulmonary disease (COPD)
Asthma	Bronchiectasis
Pulmonary embolus	Cystic fibrosis
Pulmonary oedema	Chest wall disorders

Box 2.1 Causes of acidosis.

Respiratory
- Poor gas exchange due to disease
- Depressed respiratory centre causing hypoventilation

Metabolic
- Ingestion of too much alcohol (acetaldehyde → acetic acid)
- Excessive loss of bicarbonate (e.g. severe diarrhoea)
- Increased lactic acid (e.g. exercise, shock, starvation, ketones)
- Renal failure due to excess hydrogen not being eliminated

low potassium or phosphate levels. Although the respiratory rate initially rises, the respiratory centre is able to adapt to the increasing levels of carbon dioxide, and respiratory effort gradually becomes depressed (Watson, 2000). Acute carbon dioxide retention will cause a decrease in pH (acidosis) and manifest as symptoms of confusion, lethargy, stupor, drowsiness and finally coma which may be fatal due to the presence of severe acidosis.

Respiratory failure caused by chronic lung conditions may be slower to develop, resulting from gradual deterioration of the underlying condition. Therefore patients often have fewer symptoms of carbon dioxide retention due to the physiological compensation to the raised carbon dioxide. This mechanism involves retention of bicarbonate, and in chronic respiratory failure may cause desensitisation of the central chemoreceptors. Thus chronic respiratory acidosis is compensated by a metabolic response which normalises pH levels (7.35–7.45). However, when an acute exacerbation is the cause of the deterioration this can result in acute on chronic respiratory failure which will produce a sudden increase in carbon dioxide and decrease in pH. In these circumstances there is insufficient time for metabolic compensation to occur which will result in uncharacteristic irritability, disorientation and hypotension.

Non-pulmonary causes

There are several causes of non-pulmonary respiratory acidosis (Box 2.1), including drugs such as morphine and barbiturates. This is because these drugs can affect central drive, resulting in the ability of the respiratory centre to respond to changes in the level of carbon dioxide. This central drive can also be affected by stroke, trauma, tumours or infection. The respiratory centre regulates the action of the respiratory muscles via signals transmitted through the nerves. Any damage to this conduction pathway will result in reduced ventilation and respiratory acidosis, as the ability of the respiratory muscles to respond is reduced. This could be caused by spinal cord damage, damage to the phrenic nerves and any disease which affects neurotransmission, such as motor neurone disease. As with other muscle groups, respiratory muscles are dependent on sufficient electrolyte concentrations to function optimally, in particular, potassium and phosphate (Abelow, 1998).

Metabolic acidosis

Metabolic acidosis results from a significant fall in plasma bicarbonate concentration. This is usually caused by an increase in endogenous acid production, notably lactic acid. Lactic acid is a by-product of anaerobic respiration, used by the cells when oxygen is not available. Any cause of circulatory failure which results in reduced tissue perfusion can stimulate anaerobic respiration and the production of lactic acid (Heuther, 1998). Renal failure can affect the kidney's ability to excrete acid and so can lead to metabolic acidosis. As well as reabsorbing bicarbonate, the kidney also excretes ammonium which is used for regenerating bicarbonate. These functions are compromised by renal failure. In an attempt to restore acid–base balance, the respiratory system stimulates deep, rapid respirations to expel carbon dioxide (Kussmaul respiration). Severe acidosis can lead to dysrhythmias and coma. Metabolic acidosis can be caused by anything which compromises kidney function or rapidly increases metabolic acid production. These include acute renal failure, diabetic keto-acidosis and poor tissue perfusion (Box 2.1).

Respiratory alkalosis

Respiratory alkalosis is caused by an excessive loss of carbon dioxide (Box 2.2) and is usually caused by hyperventilation. Hyperventilation can be triggered by hypoxaemia, which in turn can be exacerbated by pulmonary disease or congestive heart failure. Arterial hypoxaemia is detected by the central chemoreceptors in the aortic arch and carotid bodies. Psychological factors such as anxiety or pain may lead to tachypnoea which will produce hyperventilation (Shuldham, 1998). As the respiratory rate increases the oxygenation of arterial blood rises and there is a corresponding drop in carbon dioxide. Other causes include anaemia and prolonged or severe hypotension resulting in poor tissue

---

Box 2.2   Causes of alkalosis.

Respiratory
- Hyperventilation due to anxiety, pain and hypoxaemia
- Brain tumour/injury due to abnormal respiratory control

Metabolic
- Vomiting of acidic contents of stomach
- Intake of excessive antacids
- Severe constipation – too much HCO_3^- reabsorbed via colon

perfusion. Symptoms of respiratory alkalosis may manifest as tachyp-noea, dizziness, sweating, tingling in toes and fingers, muscle cramps and seizures.

Metabolic alkalosis

Metabolic alkalosis occurs when plasma bicarbonate is increased (Box 2.2). This can be caused by an excessive loss of metabolic acids, such as vomiting. If plasma potassium levels fall, cellular potassium is released to maintain plasma concentrations. Intracellular bicarbonate may leave the cells with the potassium. This causes an intracellular acidosis result-ing in the conservation of bicarbonate by the renal cells. Nasogastric drainage or use of diuretics is associated with metabolic alkalosis. Metabolic alkalosis is also associated with volume depletion. Loss of circulating volume leads to lowered blood pressure. This stimulates the renin–angiotensin cycle which increases plasma aldosterone. The presence of angiotensin increases bicarbonate reabsorption.

Compensation

Compensation is a mechanism whereby buffering systems work together to restore or maintain acid–base balance. For example, if meta-bolic acidosis develops, the respiratory system will increase respiration to reduce carbon dioxide levels, thereby reducing acidity. Alternatively, if respiratory acidosis develops, the renal system will alter bicarbonate levels to restore acid–base balance. While the respiratory system is quick to compensate, the metabolic system may take 24–48 hours. The speed and success of compensation can also depend on the severity of the acid–base disturbance and the acute or chronic nature of its cause.

When an acid–base imbalance occurs due to inadequate functioning of the buffering systems (kidneys or lungs) the other system attempts to compensate.

- Lungs compensate for metabolic acid–base imbalances.
- The kidneys compensate for respiratory acid–base imbalances.

Table 2.2 summarises the changes in pH, $PaCO_2$ and bicarbonate levels when acidosis and alkalosis occurs due to metabolic or respiratory causes.

Table 2.2 Summary of acid–base balance.

	Respiratory acidosis	Metabolic acidosis	Respiratory alkalosis	Metabolic alkalosis
pH	↓	↓	↑	↑
$PaCO_2$	↑	↓	↓	↑
HCO_3^-	↑	↓	↓	↑

Non-invasive monitoring for respiratory failure

Pulse oximetry

Pulse oximetry is commonly used as part of respiratory monitoring and assessment. It measures oxygen saturation by differentiating between oxygenated haemoglobin and haemoglobin with reduced oxygen (Moore, 2004). The saturation is displayed as a percentage, in addition to which, visual waveform displays can indicate the accuracy of the reading. Oxygen saturation is measured by a probes which is attached to a well-perfused area, such as a finger or earlobe; the probe can be re-usable or disposable. There are many types of probes available, all of which contain a light sensor that can determine the percentage of haemoglobin saturated with oxygen. Probes should be used on the area of the body that they are designed for in order to give accurate results, for example, a finger probe placed on an earlobe (if peripheral perfusion in the fingers is poor) may give a falsely high reading. Manufacturers guidelines regarding use of equipment should be followed to ensure accuracy of monitoring (Moore, 2004).

The indications for using pulse oximetry include monitoring the effectiveness of oxygen therapy or other respiratory support such as NIV and CPAP. Advantages of pulse oximetry are:

- It is non-invasive.
- It accurately reflects oxygenation status.
- It provides continuous information and detects changes quickly.
- It is easy to use with minimal equipment training.
- Alarms can alert staff to changes in patient status.

Pulse oximetry gives a continuous assessment of the patient's condition, unlike arterial blood gas analysis, which provides information for a specific point in time and may need to be done, potentially delaying the diagnosis of the problem. However, there are limitations in the use

> **Box 2.3 Causes of inaccurate reading of pulse oximetry.**
>
> - Poor perfusion/vasoconstriction
> - Weak pulse
> - Dysrhythmias
> - Motion artefact (e.g. restlessness or shivering)
> - Nail polish
> - Severe hypoxaemia
> - High levels of carboxyhaemoglobin (e.g. in smokers)
> - Skin pigmentation
> - Anaemia
> - High bilirubin blood levels
> - Exposure to carbon monoxide
> - Intravenous dyes

pulse oximetry and its accuracy can be affected by the factors listed in Box 2.3.

Although pulse oximetry has many advantages it is not suitable in isolation, particularly when managing acutely ill respiratory patients or those requiring oxygen therapy, NIV or CPAP, as it does not provide information about other respiratory parameters, particularly carbon dioxide and pH. Furthermore, if patients require continuous monitoring caution needs to be taken, as if the probe is too tight or left in position too long, skin damage may occur (Dougherty & Lister, 2004).

Relationship between SpO_2 and PaO_2: oxygen dissociation curve

The oxygen dissociation curve (Figure 2.1) provides important information about the relationship between the circulating partial pressure of oxygen (PaO_2) in the blood and oxygen saturation levels (SaO_2). It shows that the relationship between SaO_2 and PaO_2 is not linear and an understanding of this relationship is vital in the interpretation of oxygen saturation levels. At PaO_2 levels higher than 10.5 kPa there is little change in the SaO_2 (relating to the flat part of the curve) while below this level there is a significant fall in SaO_2 and therefore oxygen content (steep part of the curve).

The oxygen dissociation curve shows the equilibrium of oxyhaemoglobin and non-bonded haemoglobin and indicates the per cent saturation of haemoglobin at various partial pressures of oxygen.

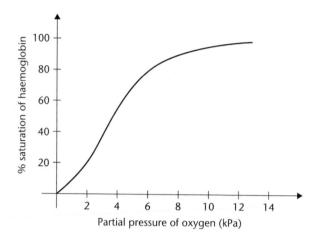

Figure 2.1   Oxygen dissociation curve.

Haemoglobin binds to oxygen to form oxyhaemoglobin at high partial pressures of oxygen, usually in the lungs. At full saturation, all the erythrocytes are in the form of oxyhaemoglobin; as the erythrocytes reach tissues lacking oxygen, there will be a fall in partial pressure of oxygen, and oxyhaemoglobin releases the oxygen to form haemoglobin (Schmidt-Nielsen, 1997).

The oxygen dissociation curve is sigmoid shaped as a result of the binding of oxygen to the four polypeptide chains: haemoglobin is more attracted to oxygen when three of the four polypeptide chains are bound to oxygen. Three factors influence the binding of oxygen: temperature, pH and organic phosphate levels. Shifts to the right are caused by an increase in temperature (i.e. pyrexia), a decrease in pH (by addition of carbon dioxide or other acids as in acidosis and hypercapnia) or an increase in 2,3-diphosphoglycerate (DPG) which is the primary organic phosphate in mammals. This results in a lower SaO_2 for the same PaO_2 as the affinity of oxygen and for haemoglobin is decreased, to allow easier unloading at the tissues. Shifts to the left are caused by alkalosis, hypocapnia and falls in body temperature resulting in a higher SaO_2 for the same PaO_2 as the affinity of oxygen for haemoglobin is increased, resulting in tighter binding of oxygen and haemoglobin, with more difficulty in unloading oxygen at the tissues.

Transcutaneous monitoring

Oxygen and carbon dioxide pressures can be measured transcutaneously using electrodes combined with sensors (Williams, 1998). The electrodes heat the skin allowing diffusion from vasodilated vessels, which in neonates is accurate due to the skin being thin and well vascularised. However, in adults there are often wide discrepancies between arterial and transcutaneous blood gas measurements (Rosner et al., 1999), with transcutaneous carbon dioxide levels often being higher than those measured arterially. This method of non-invasive monitoring is therefore only suitable for monitoring trends in stable patients, for example in sleep studies.

Invasive monitoring for respiratory failure

Arterial blood gas sampling

Arterial blood gas samples are taken to determine arterial concentrations of oxygen and carbon dioxide and provide additional information on the acid–base balance through detecting levels of pH, bicarbonate and base excess, to aid diagnosis. Most arterial blood gas analysers can also provide electrolyte levels, including lactate. These values are important when evaluating the clinical status of deteriorating patients or to determine the response to interventions, such as NIV (Middleston et al., 2006). Arterial blood gas samples may be taken when respiratory failure is suspected to establish levels of carbon dioxide and oxygen allowing a distinction to be made between Type I and Type II respiratory failure. Arterial blood gas analysis can also assist with diagnosis of renal failure and diabetic ketoacidosis by establishing acid–base balance.

All samples need to be collected into a heparinised syringe to avoid clotting of the sample which will alter the results and potentially damage the analyser. A variety of prepared heparinised syringes are available, which are designed to suit the method employed for obtaining the sample. Frequency of sampling will depend on the clinical need of the patient, changes to interventions or treatment and the willingness of the patient to undergo the procedures discussed later in the book. Verbal consent needs to be obtained, and the reasons for the sample being taken explained so the patient understands the need for the investigation. There are three ways of obtaining blood samples for blood gas analysis:

- Indwelling arterial catheter (arterial lines)
- Single puncture of the artery (arterial 'stab')
- Capillary earlobe blood samples (earlobe gases)

Arterial lines

Indwelling arterial lines allow samples to be taken without additional pain and discomfort, and are usually only used in intensive care and high dependency units (Woodrow, 2004). This is due to the risk of unde-tected disconnection and the risk of infection. In addition, accidental injection leading to arterial spasm, peripheral vessel damage and local damage to the artery can occur (Dougherty & Lister, 2004). Signs of such damage include pain and cooling of the peripheries. Change in appear-ance of the peripheries when the cannula is flushed, such as mottling or blanching, is another sign of potential damage (Dougherty & Lister, 2004). In order to avoid permanent damage, the cannula may have to be removed (Adams & Osborne, 2005). Healthcare professionals require compet-ence in managing the arterial line and obtaining a sample safely. All techniques involving the manipulation of the cannula must be aseptic.

Indwelling arterial lines need to be kept patent, usually by continuous pressure applied through a specialised pressurised giving set containing fluid, usually saline (Figure 2.2). This is to avoid the risk of clots forming on the end of the catheter which can enter the general circulation. In order to obtain accurate results, this fluid needs to be removed before the sample is obtained to prevent the sample being contaminated by dilution. In an attempt to reduce blood loss among critically ill patients, the volume removed from indwelling arterial catheters prior to obtaining the sample has traditionally been the volume of the dead space (usually 2 ml). However, a number of studies have demonstrated that results

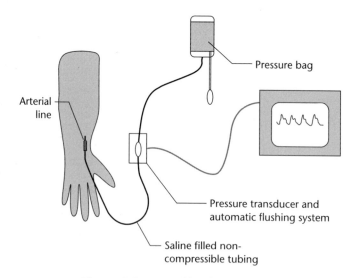

Arterial line

Pressure bag

Pressure transducer and automatic flushing system

Saline filled non-compressible tubing

Figure 2.2   Arterial line/pressure bag.

obtained from samples can vary according to the discard volume taken. Rickard et al. (2003) recommended a discard volume of twice the dead space to ensure accurate results.

Arterial 'stabs'

An arterial 'stab' involves taking blood with a syringe and needle from an artery, most commonly from the radial artery, although the femoral can also be used. The process can be painful because arteries are deeper than veins and for this reason a local anaesthetic may be administered to the site prior to the procedure (Woodrow, 2004). Prior to a radial arterial 'stab', an Allen's test should be performed (Royal College of Surgeons, 2006). This test checks blood flow to the hand. In the event of arterial spasm, blood flow to peripheries will be reduced. Allen's test (Figure 2.3) involves compressing the radial artery until blanching of the skin occurs. This usually takes several seconds. Skin colour should return to normal within 10–14 seconds of the pressure being released. If skin colour is normal within this time frame, Allen's test is positive and arterial 'stab' can be performed. If Allen's test is negative, arterial 'stab' must not take place as this indicates inadequate circulation. An alternative site for arterial 'stab' must be identified (e.g. femoral artery).

When obtaining the sample the needle should be inserted into the artery under aseptic conditions at an angle (Figure 2.4). There are two ways to aspirate the blood. One is to insert the needle through the artery until bone is reached and then withdraw the needle while aspirating until blood flows into the syringe. Alternatively, complete puncture of

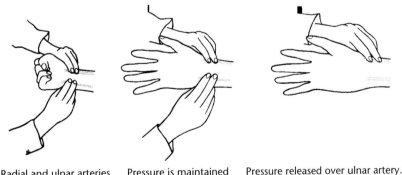

Radial and ulnar arteries obstructed while patient clenches fist

Pressure is maintained over radial and ulnar arteries while patient gently opens hand

Pressure released over ulnar artery. The palm should turn pink, indicating that collateral flow is adequate (positive Allen's test)

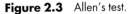

Figure 2.3 Allen's test.

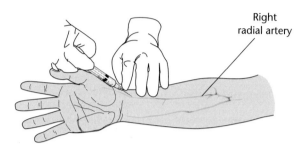

Figure 2.4   Arterial 'stab'.

the artery can be avoided by penetrating the tissues until the artery is reached. Once the sample has been obtained, pressure must be applied to the puncture site for at least 2 minutes to avoid blood leaking into the tissues and forming a haematoma. This will reduce pain and preserve the availability of sites for future sample collection.

Earlobe gases

Taking an arterialised capillary earlobe blood sample is associated with fewer complications and this procedure is often more accepted by patients as it is less painful than an arterial 'stab'. This technique is particularly useful for assessing the need for long-term oxygen therapy (LTOT) and also for assessing the response to NIV. As this technique is less painful (Dar et al., 1995) than arterial 'stabs', the frequent need for assessment will be less distressing and can produce accurate results (Pitkin et al., 1994). There is evidence to suggest that although the technique has been used to obtain blood samples for many years (Wimpress et al., 2005), it is under-used in adult clinical practice (Ugramurthy et al., 2004). The technique has been adopted by some for the evaluation of chronic respiratory conditions such as chronic obstructive pulmonary disease (Murphy et al., 2006). It has also been utilised for the assessment of those requiring LTOT (Eaton et al., 2001).

Prior to taking the sample, the earlobe is coated with nicotinate cream to cause vasodilation. This will result in the earlobe feeling unusually warm. When the sample is to be taken, all traces of the cream must be removed and the earlobe supported with a rubber bung. The stab should be made close to the tip of the pinna, the first drops of blood removed with gauze and blood collection should be free flowing allowing quick collection into a thin glass capillary tube by surface tension (Figure 2.5). The presence of air bubbles in the tube necessitates the drawing of a new sample. The sample should be analysed immediately.

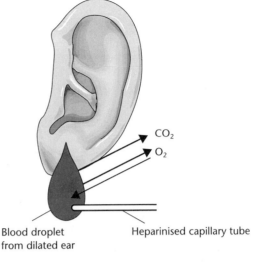

CO$_2$

O$_2$

Blood droplet
from dilated ear

Heparinised capillary tube

Figure 2.5 Earlobe sampling.

The sample site should be covered with gauze and held firmly until bleeding stops. When bleeding has stopped, a plaster can then be applied to the area. A good technique is required in order to obtain accurate results. Table 2.3 outlines the procedure and the rationale for taking capillary earlobe gases and Figure 2.6 illustrates the areas of competence that are required.

Table 2.3 Procedure for obtaining arterialised blood gas sample.

Preparation	Rationale
The procedure is explained to the patient	To obtain the patient's consent to the procedure
It is important to enquire if patient is taking any anticoagulants (warfarin, aspirin)	**It may be necessary to make a smaller cut to avoid haemorrhage**
A paper towel is placed on patient's shoulder	To protect the patient's clothing if blood spilled
The front and back of the earlobe is liberally coated with nicotinate cream, which is left on for at least 10 minutes to induce vasodilation. The patient is informed that the ear will become warm	Important to vasodilate and arterialise ear well, to encourage a good blood supply
The patient is asked to remain seated during the waiting period, when resting gases are required. They are also warned to take care and not touch the cream and that if it gets onto their hands, they should inform the technician so that their hands can be washed	To give an appropriate result for resting gases The cream may cause irritation if it enters the eyes

Table 2.3   (continued)

Method	Rationale
Wear gloves	Reduce the risk of blood contamination as per standard precautions
Wipe cream off well and massage ear to increase blood flow	Failure to remove all the cream can affect the pH of the blood
With a rubber bung to support the back of the earlobe, make a stab close to the tip of the pinna. The short distance from the stab to the tip of the pinna allows drops of blood to form quickly and reduces the chance of smearing. Wipe away the first drop of blood with gauze	If the cut is too high it will smear and make collection difficult, which will result in oxygenation of the blood The first drop of blood may be diluted by tissue fluid
The blood flow is usually adequate but sometimes it is necessary to pierce through the earlobe to the other side. **The blood should be free flowing** and collected as quickly as possible from the centre of the droplet	To reduce the risk of room air contamination
The blood is drawn into a thin glass capillary tube by surface tension under the control of a gloved finger over the open end of the tube. To regulate the blood flow, move the capillary distal to the earlobe downwards to increase the flow or upwards to decrease the flow rate	To ensure adequate filling of the capillary tube
If air bubbles enter the capillary tube, wipe the earlobe and start again, allowing the first supply to drop onto the tissue. If this is too difficult, use a new capillary tube. If the ear bleeds slowly, wipe and massage with a gauze swab. The ear should not be squeezed. If this does not help, another cut may be necessary	Avoid squeezing/milking the area as this may lead to de-arterialisation of the blood, haemolysis of blood cells, admixture of blood and tissue fluid
After collection of the blood, put a clean gauze swab on the ear and ask the patient to hold it firmly. Close both ends of the tube with your fingers (if the analyser is close by) or with two rubber stoppers, and aspirate into analyser without delay. If you have not been assessed to use the analyser, ensure other staff are available to run the sample through analyser without delay	To ensure safe transfer of sample and reduce the risk of room air contamination Training to use the blood gas analyser is necessary for both the quality of the results and efficient working of the equipment
A dry swab is held to the ear by the patient until the site has stopped bleeding. A plaster is then applied to the area	To ensure site has stopped bleeding
If repeat samples are required, on some patients the prepared site may bleed freely and a second cut may not be necessary. If a second cut is required, it should be made away from the first cut to avoid bruising and scarring. This particularly applies to hospitalised patients on ventilators, from whom several samples may need to be taken over a few days, hence the ears should be alternated	
Discard sharps into rigid sharps bin, waste and blood stained gauze into yellow clinical waste bag for incineration and wash hands thoroughly	Reduce the risk of cross-infection and comply with risk and waste regulations

	Competency Assessment for Performing Capillary Earlobe Blood Gases	Yes	No

Name: .... Title: ....

	Critical performance observations	Yes	No
1	Has carried out training on the use of blood gas analyser and has passcode.		
2	Identifies the indications for obtaining CBG.		
3	Verifies patient details, selects correct equipment, washes hands, positions patient correctly.		
4	Explains procedure to patient, and questions patient regarding anticoagulant drugs.		
5	Assesses site and applies vasodilator cream with gloved finger correctly.		
6	Waits for appropriate time and takes arterialised sample: a) Performs correct stab to the pinna and ensures blood flow is adequate. b) Disposes blade correctly. c) Wipes first drop of blood with swab. d) Takes sample speedily, without smearing, and without milking the ear. e) Ensures there are no air bubbles in sample. f) Asks patient to apply pressure to site with gauze while capping sample. g) Applies plaster to the site. h) Sample is processed via blood gas analyser without delay.		
7	Washes hands, reassesses patient and completes documentation.		
8	States the normal range for ABG results, and correlates results with patient's status.		

Number	Date	Assessed by (please sign)	Print name
1			
2			
3			
4			
5			
6			
7			
8			
9			
10			

Comments:	Outcome: Successful ☐ Unsuccessful ☐

The above healthcare professional has knowledge and understanding of the theory of capillary earlobe blood gas sampling and has been witnessed on at least ten occasions undertaking the procedure correctly.

Signature of assessor: _____

Designation: _____ Date: _____

Figure 2.6 Competency assessment for performing capillary earlobe blood gases.

Sample analysis

Once the sample has been taken, the accuracy of the results will be affected by how it is handled (Woodrow, 2004). Delaying the analysis of samples will affect results due to the continued gas exchange and metabolism of blood cells. It is recommended that samples should be analysed as quickly as possible and should not remain at room temperature for more than 15 minutes (Beaumont, 1997). Storing the sample in ice can prolong the reliability of the sample, but can also cause haemolysis, causing inaccurate results (Woodrow, 2004). Air bubbles in the sample can also affect accuracy of the results and should be expelled immediately. Delayed processing of the sample can also allow blood cells and plasma to separate. This is why samples are mixed during transportation by rolling the syringe. Shaking should be avoided as this may damage the cells. All machines have their own method of operation and it is important for accuracy that they are used correctly and maintained in accordance with manufacturers recommendations. The option to interpret results specific to the temperature is sometimes required as this can affect the results. If using this method, it is important to ensure consistency of the temperature measurement. Temperature will vary between measurement sites, for example axilla and tympanic, and inaccurate recording of temperature through poor technique will also affect results. Some clinicians, therefore, prefer to measure all samples at 37°C to ensure consistency (Woodrow, 2004). It is important that all measurements of arterial blood gases in a clinical area follow the same method, whichever method is used.

Interpretation of blood gases

Blood gas analysers produce a printed report of the analysis. Inclusions in the report will depend on the machine used; values for electrolytes, e.g. potassium and sodium, are common, as are glucose and haemoglobin levels. The usual unit of measurement for carbon dioxide and oxygen levels in the UK is kiloPascals (kPa); in the USA, measurements are expressed in millimetres of mercury (mmHg). Blood gas interpretation will allow acid–base balance to be determined and whether the patient is in Type I or Type II respiratory failure. To determine this, the following need to be interpreted in relation to normal (Box 2.4) and the patient's baseline values:

- pH (potential hydrogen) – measures acidity or alkalinity
- $PaCO_2$
- PaO_2
- HCO_3
- Base excess (BE) (measurement of the number of moles of acid or base required to return 1 litre of blood to pH 7.4)

Box 2.4   Normal blood gas values.

Value	Normal range
pH	7.35–7.45
$PaCO_2$	4.5–6.0 kPa
PaO_2	11.5–13.5 kPa
HCO_3	22–26 mmol
BE	+2 to –2

A systematic interpretation of the results is required:

1. Is the patient acidotic or alkalotic, or is the pH normal? An abnormal pH suggests either that the problem is new, or that a longer standing problem has become decompensated.
   a. When the pH is abnormal, if the direction of change of the carbon dioxide explains the abnormality seen in pH then this is a primary respiratory problem.
   b. When the pH is abnormal and the direction of change is not explained by the carbon dioxide, but is explained by the direction of change in bicarbonate then this is a primary metabolic problem.
2. Is there a partial compensatory change in the other parameter (bicarbonate if pH explained by carbon dioxide, carbon dioxide if the pH explained by bicarbonate)?
3. If the pH is normal, is this a fully compensated acid–base disturbance manifest by abnormalities of both carbon dioxide and bicarbonate?
4. Finally, what is the PaO_2 and how does this relate to the fraction of inspired oxygen (FiO_2)?

When recording the blood gas results it is important that it is noted if they were taken on air or oxygen, as this will allow an accurate interpretation.

Case studies

Case study 2.1   Pneumonia

Jack is admitted to hospital with pneumonia initially in Type II respiratory failure. Due to severe dyspnoea he becomes exhausted resulting in deterioration due to being unable to maintain adequate ventilation. He is coughing but is not able to produce any sputum. He has been previously fit and well. He is given 60% oxygen. His blood gases are:

pH	7.3
$PaCO_2$	7.45 kPa
PaO_2	6.8 kPa
HCO_3^-	26 mmol
Base excess	+2.3
SaO_2	87%

The pH indicates an acidotic picture. The carbon dioxide level is high, whilst the bicarbonate and base excess are within normal limits. Jack therefore has a respiratory acidosis with no metabolic compensation. This would indicate a recent problem as metabolic compensation would only be present after 2–3 days.

Case study 2.2   Hyperventilation syndrome

Cindy has recently been diagnosed with hyperventilation syndrome. She is admitted to the emergency department after being found collapsed by her mother. On arrival, she has a respiratory rate of 36/minute and is distressed. Her blood gases on room air are:

pH	7.49
$PaCO_2$	3.35 kPa
PaO_2	14.1 kPa
HCO_3^-	22 mmol
Base excess	+2.3
SaO_2	98%

The pH indicates an alkalotic picture. The carbon dioxide level is low, while the oxygen, bicarbonate, base excess are within normal limits. Cindy therefore has a respiratory alkalosis with no metabolic compensation. On questioning she describes dizziness and tingling of her hands, toes and lips. Once her respiratory rate has returned to normal, her symptoms and alkalosis normalise. She is referred to physiotherapy for treatment of her hyperventilation.

Case study 2.3   COPD: Type II respiratory failure with compensation

Muriel has a confirmed diagnosis of chronic obstructive pulmonary disease and her forced expiratory volume in 1 second (FEV_1) is less that 30% predicted indicting that she has severe disease. She is on LTOT at home and following a viral infection, is admitted to hospital for treatment of her acute exacerbation. Her blood gases on 2 l/min oxygen are:

pH	7.29
$PaCO_2$	9.45 kPa
PaO_2	5.8 kPa
HCO_3^-	31 mmol
Base excess	+3.3
SaO_2	83%

The pH indicates an acidotic picture. The carbon dioxide level is high, along with raised bicarbonate and base excess. Muriel therefore has a respiratory acidosis with metabolic compensation. She is treated with oxygen and NIV.

References

Abelow, B. (1998) *Understanding Acid Base*. Williams and Wilkins, Philadelphia, London.

Adams, S.K. & Osborne, S. (2005) Monitoring the critically ill patient. In *Critical Care Nursing: Science and Practice*, 2nd edn. Chapter 5. Oxford University Press. Oxford.

Beaumont, T. (1997) How to guides: arterial blood gas sampling. *Care of the Critically Ill*, **13**, 1, centre insert.

Cooper, N. (2004) Acute care: arterial blood gases. *British Medical Journal*, **12**, 89–132.

Dar, K., Williams, T., Aitken, R., Woods, K.L. & Fletcher, S. (1995) Arterial versus capillary sampling for analysing blood gas pressures. *British Medical Journal*, **310**, 24–25.

Dougherty, L. & Lister, S. (eds) (2004) *The Royal Marsden Hospital Manual of Clinical Nursing Procedures*, 6th edn. Blackwell, Oxford.

Eaton, T., Rudkin, S. & Garrett, J.E. (2001) The clinical utility of arterialized earlobe capillary blood in the assessment of patients for long-term oxygen therapy. *Respiratory Medicine*, **95**, 655–660.

Huether, S. (1998) Alterations of pulmonary function. In: McNance, K.L. & Huether, S. (eds) *Pathophysiology: the Biologic Basis for Disease in Adults and Children*, 3rd edn. Mosby, St Louis.

Middleston, P., Kelly, A.M., Brown, J. & Robertson, M. (2006) Agreement between arterial and central venous values for pH, bicarbonate, base excess and lactate. *Emergency Medicine Journal*, **23**, 622–624.

Moore, T. (2004) Pulse oximetry. In: *High Dependency Nursing Care* (eds T. Moore & P. Woodrow). Routledge, London.

Murphy, R., Thethy, S., Raby, S., Beckley, J., Terrace, J. & Fiddler, C. (2006) Capillary blood gases in acute exacerbations of COPD. *Respiratory Medicine,* **100** (4), 682–686.

Pitkin, A.D., Roberts, C.M. & Wedzicha, J.A. (1994) Arterialized earlobe gas analysis. An underused technique. *Thorax,* **49**, 364–366.

Rickard, C., Couchman, B., Schmidt, S., Dank, A. & Purdie, D. (2003) A discard volume of twice the dead space ensures clinically accurate arterial blood gases and electrolytes and prevents unnecessary blood loss. *Critical Care Medicine,* **31** (6), 1654–1658.

Rosner, V., Hannhart, B., Chabot, F. & Polu, J.M. (1999) Validity of trans- cutaneous oxygen/carbon dioxide pressure measurement in the monitoring of mechanical ventilation in stable chronic respiratory failure. *European Respiratory Journal,* **13**, 1044–1047.

Royal College of Surgeons (2006) Arterial blood gases for the surgical trainee – when, how and what does it mean? Available at: www.edu.rcsed.ac.uk/ lectures (accessed 17 May 2008).

Schmidt-Nielsen, K. (1997) *Animal Physiology: Adaptation and Environment.* Cambridge University Press, Cambridge.

Shuldham, C. (ed.) (1998) *Cardiorespiratory Nursing.* Stanley Thornes, Kingston upon Thames.

Ugramurthy, S., Rathna, N., Naik, S.D. & Kurtkoti, S. (2004) Comparative study of blood gas and acid base parameters of capillary with arterial blood samples. *Indian Journal of Anaesthesia,* **48** (6), 469–471.

Watson, R. (2000) *Anatomy and Physiology for Nurses.* Bailliere Tindall, Edinburgh.

Williams, A.J. (1998) ABC of oxygen: assessing and interpreting arterial blood gases and acid–base balance. *British Medical Journal,* **317**, 1213–1216.

Wimpress, S., Vara, D. & Brightling, C. (2005) Improving the sampling technique of arterialized capillary samples to obtain more accurate PaO_2 measure- ments. *Chronic Respiratory Disease,* **2** (1), 47–50.

Woodrow, P. (2004) Arterial blood gas analysis. *Nursing Standard,* **18** (21), 45–52.

Chapter 3
OXYGEN THERAPY

Oxygen therapy is the administration of oxygen at concentrations greater than that in room air, to treat or prevent hypoxaemia and thereby increasing the availability of oxygen to the body tissues. Supplemental oxygen may be required during acute illness or as a long-term treatment for those with an underlying respiratory condition. The amount of supplemental oxygen delivered will be determined by the cause of the hypoxaemia and whether the patient has hypoxaemic (Type I) or hypercapnic (Type II) respiratory failure.

Hypoxaemic (Type I) respiratory failure

Hypoxaemic (Type I) respiratory failure is often a result of reversible, acute respiratory conditions, which include asthma, pneumonia and pulmonary embolism. In this group of patients it is necessary to initiate high concentrations of oxygen (60–100%) to prevent hypoxic tissue damage. Usually this only needs to be administered until treatments such as bronchodilators, corticosteroids and antibiotics start to improve the underlying condition. The aim of oxygen therapy for patients with Type I respiratory failure is to correct hypoxaemia to a normal or near-normal oxygen level so that the PaO_2 is above 8 kPa or more preferably >10 kPa, or when pulse oximetry is being used then the SpO_2 should be 92% or above.

Hypercapnic (Type II) respiratory failure

Hypercapnic (Type II) respiratory failure is not as easily detected, as pulse oximetry does not detect carbon dioxide levels. Therefore, further assessment, including arterial blood gas analysis is required if hypercapnic respiratory failure is suspected. Initially, while awaiting arterial blood gases a careful clinical assessment, including anticipation of patients at risk of hypercapnic respiratory failure (such as those with severe chronic obstructive pulmonary disease (COPD), bronchiectasis, cystic fibrosis or neuromuscular disorders), as well as clinical signs of carbon dioxide retention, should be used to guide oxygen therapy. Carbon dioxide is a vasodilator so patients with hypercapnia may appear flushed with dilated peripheral veins, have a bounding pulse and headache due to cranial vasodilation (Dripps & Comroe, 1947). High concentrations of carbon dioxide will alter the level of consciousness and if not treated, drowsiness and a flapping tremor will lead to coma (Refsum, 1963). Cham et al. (2002) identified that the presence of drowsiness, flushing and intercostal retraction along with the diagnosis were the best clinical predictors of hypercapnia. However, the only accurate way of identifying hypercapnic respiratory failure and its severity is by arterial blood gas analysis.

Patients with severe COPD, bronchiectasis and cystic fibrosis are at particular risk of Type II respiratory failure due to a reduced hypoxic respiratory drive and increased ventilation–perfusion mismatch. Carbon dioxide retention is more likely to occur during exacerbations which Rudolph et al. (1977) suggest is due to a difference in hypoxic ventilatory sensitivity between stable disease state and exacerbation. If high concentrations of inspired oxygen are administered to those at high risk of Type II respiratory failure this can lead to carbon dioxide retention ($PaCO_2$ > 6.0 kPa) and subsequent respiratory acidosis (pH < 7.35). Georgopolous & Anthonisen (1990) identified that it is relatively uncommon to have oxygen-induced carbon dioxide retention with a fractional concentration of inspired oxygen (FiO_2) of less than 35%. Therefore low flow oxygen (24–28%) should initially be administered and titrated upwards if arterial blood gases indicate it is necessary and can be done without causing carbon dioxide retention. Arterial blood gases should then be taken 30 minutes to an hour after commencing oxygen therapy, so that the inspired oxygen can be titrated in response to the results. The aim is to correct hypoxaemia by increasing the PaO_2 to at least 8.0 kPa or a SpO_2 of 90%, thereby preventing tissue hypoxia and secondary complication such as cor pulmonale. This may appear quite low, however, due to the shape of the dissociation curve, increasing the levels to more than 7.98 kPa provides little additional benefit, but may increase the risk of carbon dioxide retention in this group of patients (Mitrouska et al., 2006). If this cannot be achieved then additional treatments such as non-invasive ventilation need to be considered (Plant et al., 2000).

Delivery of supplemental oxygen

Two components are required to deliver supplemental oxygen therapy:

- Oxygen source – compressed, concentrated, liquid.
- Delivery device – masks, nasal cannula, transtracheal device.

Sources of oxygen

Compressed oxygen

Compressed oxygen is the most recognised source of oxygen, as once compressed it is stored under pressure within a mental cylinder. The reason for the oxygen being under pressure is so that it can be delivered without the need for electricity. There is an increased risk of fire due to the pressurisation. The cylinders come in a variety of sizes and the choice of size depends on the purpose of its use.

Liquid oxygen

Liquid oxygen is often referred to as LOX; this is where the gaseous oxygen has been converted into a liquid. Oxygen is a liquid at temperatures below its boiling point of $-183°C$, at which time it takes on a pale blue colour and takes up a tenth of the space of compressed oxygen. The liquid oxygen will convert back to gas at temperatures greater than $-118.6°C$. Therefore it must be stored in an insulated container which keeps the temperature of the oxygen at $-170°C$. Prior to the liquid oxygen being delivered to the patient it passes through a warming coil which converts the liquid back into a gas.

Concentrated oxygen

Concentrated oxygen is produced by an oxygen concentrator which runs off an electricity supply and draws in room air as a source of the oxygen. Atmospheric air consists of approximately 78% nitrogen and 21% oxygen and the aim of the concentrator is to separate these gases so that an oxygen source is available. This is achieved by use of zeolite which captures nitrogen molecules from the compressed air drawn into the machine from the atmosphere, resulting in a continuous supply of oxygen of up to a flow rate of up to 5 l/min. The accuracy of delivery depends on the pressure being maintained (see p. 64 for further explanation).

Oxygen delivery devices

Oxygen masks, nasal cannulae and transtracheal devices can be used to transfer the oxygen from the oxygen source to the lungs. Furthermore, the devices have an important role in regulating the amount of inspired oxygen that is received. Devices can be divided into two main categories:

- Fixed performance
- Variable performance

Fixed performance Venturi devices

Fixed performance Venturi devices (Figure 3.1) provide an accurate level of inspired oxygen, which are very precise between 24% and 50%. This is because the Venturi mask uses Bernoulli's principle (Mitrouska et al., 2006). The constant flow of oxygen is forced through a narrow restriction in the Venturi barrel, which causes its velocity to increase and results in room air being entrained through the holes in the side of the Venturi barrel at the point when the lateral pressure becomes sub-atmospheric (Figure 3.2). The size of the holes where the air is entrained and how much the flow of oxygen is restricted will determine how much air is mixed with the oxygen.

The Venturi mask is particularly useful for delivering controlled low flow oxygen therapy (24–28%) to patients at risk of carbon dioxide retention during acute exacerbations, including:

- Severe chronic obstructive pulmonary disease
- Severe cystic fibrosis

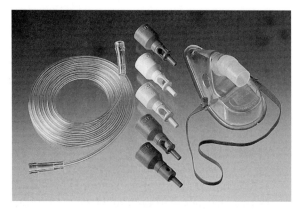

Figure 3.1 Venturi mask. With kind permission from Air Products Healthcare.

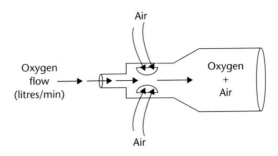

Figure 3.2 Venturi principle.

Table 3.1 Venturi mask colour coding and flow rates.

Per cent	Venturi barrel colour	Flow rate
24	Blue	2 l/min
28	White	2 l/min or 4 l or 6 l/min
31	Orange	6 l/min
35	Yellow	8 l/min
40	Red	10 l/min
60	Green	15 l/min

- Severe bronchiectasis
- Severe neuromuscular/chest wall disorders
- Morbid obesity

The Venturi devices are colour coded to match the percentages of oxygen delivery. However, this will only be achieved if the flow rate indicted on the barrel is also delivered. Table 3.1 indicates that colour coding for the different percentages and the matching flow rates. The Venturi mask allows the total gas flow rate from the mask to exceed the inspiratory flow rate of the patient. For the majority of patients this will be achieved, although Jones et al. (1984) demonstrated that patients with a respiratory rate greater than 30 breaths per minute often have an inspiratory flow rate above the minimum flow rate specified on the barrel. In these circumstances the British Thoracic Society (2008) suggests that the oxygen flow rate for the Venturi mask may need to be set 50% above the minimum flow rate listed on the barrel.

Variable performance oxygen devices

Variable performance devices are less accurate as the amount of inspired oxygen delivered will vary, depending on the rate and depth of respirations. There are different types of variable performance devices,

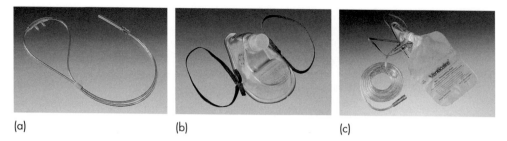

(a)   (b)   (c)

Figure 3.3 Variable performance devices. (a) Nasal cannulae. (b) Simple mask. (c) Non-rebreathing mask. With kind permission from Air Products Healthcare.

designed to deliver either low- or high-flow oxygen. The most commonly used ones are:

- Nasal cannulae
- Simple masks (i.e. 'Hudson' mask)
- Non-rebreathing mask

Nasal cannulae (Figure 3.3a) are designed to deliver low- to medium-flow oxygen once the patient's condition has stabilised and are often more accepted by patients as they are less claustrophobic, do not impede communication and allow the patient to eat and drink while receiving oxygen therapy. Waldau and colleagues' (1998) evaluation of oxygen delivery devices demonstrated that nasal cannulae at 1–4 l/min are approximately equivalent to 24–40% oxygen from Venturi masks. Although the oxygen dose continues to rise up to flows of 6 l/min it is not usually tolerated by patients, as at flow rates above 4 l/min via nasal cannulae, the patient experiences discomfort and nasal dryness (Waldau et al., 1998). If a patient is a mouth breather, oxygen delivery may be impaired (Kory et al., 1962; Gibson et al., 1976). However, the American Thoracic Society COPD guidelines (2004) suggest that nasal oxygen delivery is still beneficial in mouth breathers since only a small nasal inspiratory flow is necessary, and some oxygen is stored in the nasal and sinus passages. Provided that the patient has been assessed while using nasal cannulae and is monitored using pulse oximetry, there is no reason why nasal cannulae cannot be used for mouth breathers. The two prongs of the nasal cannulae are curved and should be placed in the nostril downwards so the oxygen is directed towards the airway. The nasal cannulae are held in place by looping the tubing around the ear but care needs to be taken as pressure sores can develop behind the ear, so regular inspection is required and if redness is present padding may be required.

If high levels of inspiratory oxygen are indicated, a simple mask (Figure 3.3b), such as the Hudson mask, is suitable to deliver 40–60%. Serious illnesses requiring moderate to high levels of supplemental oxygen to correct hypoxaemia include:

- Acute asthma
- Pneumonia
- Acute heart failure
- Pulmonary embolism
- Pleural effusions
- Advanced pulmonary fibrosis/interstitial lung disease
- Severe anaemia
- Sickle cell crisis

If there is an insufficient response to 40–60% oxygen then high-flow oxygen should be initiated and other treatments, such as continuous positive airway pressure (CPAP) and ventilation, considered if indicated.

For delivery of high inspiratory oxygen levels of up to 90%, a non-rebreathing mask with reservoir bag and a one-way valve is suitable (Figure 3.3c). Critical illnesses requiring high levels of supplemental oxygen to correct hypoxaemia include:

- Cardiac arrest or resuscitation
- Shock sepsis
- Major trauma
- Near-drowning
- Anaphylaxis
- Major pulmonary haemorrhage
- Major head injury
- Carbon monoxide poisoning

Patients requiring high-flow oxygen are critically ill and therefore need to be cared for in a high dependency care environment as many of these patients may need to be intubated.

Variable performance masks are not designed to function with low-flow oxygen as it has been demonstrated by Jensen et al. (1991) that flow rates of less than 5 l/min can cause an increased resistance to breathing which may result in the build-up of carbon dioxide within the mask and which may be re-breathed. It has also been suggested that high concentrations of oxygen (>60%) administered to patients for a prolonged period may cause lung damage as high concentrations of oxygen will encourage collapse of alveoli with low ventilation perfusion ratios. In practice there is little evidence to support this, and it should not prevent its use in treating severe hypoxia as the consequence of tissue hypoxia is likely to be catastrophic. However, if high inspiratory flows are required for prolonged periods, other treatments such as high-flow CPAP should be considered.

Transtracheal oxygen

Transtracheal oxygen is delivered through a small flexible plastic catheter which is percutaneously placed directly into the trachea through an opening in the neck between the second and third tracheal rings. As the oropharynx is bypassed the dead space is reduced which results in lower oxygen flow rates being required to correct hypoxaemia. Compared with nasal cannula, Hoffman et al. (1991) showed that transtracheal oxygen flow rates were reduced by 50% at rest and 30% on exertion. The other advantage is that the oxygen tubing is less visible which may increase the adherence with oxygen therapy, particularly ambulatory oxygen as when the patient leaves the home they are likely to be less self-conscious. However, transtracheal oxygen is not without complications. These include catheter blockage by mucus, catheter displacement, cellulitis, subcutaneous emphysema, haemoptysis and severed catheter. To prevent mucous balls accumulating and blocking the catheter a daily cleaning regimen and frequent catheter changes need to be performed, which increases the care compared with someone receiving oxygen via nasal cannulae. If the catheter does get blocked, it needs to be changed immediately as the patient will not be receiving their prescribed oxygen. Kampelmacher et al. (1997) demonstrated that transtracheal oxygen can be delivered safely provided that patients are carefully selected. Therefore a risk assessment needs to be carried out; contraindications that exclude patients using this route for oxygen delivery include inability to practise self-care, subglottic stenosis, vocal cord paralysis and coagulation disorders. Patients at high risk of complications may be on high-dose steroids (e.g. prednisone 30 mg), have diabetes, connective tissue disease and severe obesity.

Humidification

Oxygen may need to be humidified to counteract its drying effect and is usually used with high flow rates, usually greater than 4 l/min, or during acute infective exacerbations. There are different ways of humidifying oxygen:

- Heated humidifier systems
- Large-volume nebulisation systems
- Heat and moisture exchange systems

Heated humidifier systems

These work by passing the oxygen through a heated sterile water system (e.g. Fisher Paykel heated humidifier, REMstar Heated Humidifier). These systems work on the principle that warming the gas increases its capacity to hold water vapour, whereas cooling it reduces its capacity to hold water vapour. The mucociliary transport system works at its maximum rate when inspired gases are conditioned to 37°C, which means that there is 100% relative humidity or an absolute humidity of 44 mg water vapour per litre of air. Although these systems are the most efficient at providing humidification they are also the most expensive. They are usually used when the nasopharynx has been by-passed, as in the case of someone with a tracheostomy.

Large-volume nebulisation systems

These systems (e.g. Respiflo system) work on the principle of converting water into an aerosol so that particles are small enough to reach the respiratory tract to loosen thickened secretions and ensure the mucociliary escalator functions correctly. These systems are usually used in patients requiring high flow rates (>4 l/min) or in those having difficulty clearing respiratory secretions.

Ultrasonic nebulisation is a super-saturation nebuliser system that uses ultrasonic passing through water to produce a dense aerosol which can rapidly hydrate the respiratory tract. Due to the density of the aerosol, bronchospasm is sometimes experienced. Both these systems can be delivered either using cold or heated water, although a heated system will provide greater humidity.

Heat and moisture exchange filters

Heat and moisture exchange filters are used in tracheostomised patients, as in these patients the nasopharynx is by-passed, which affects the body's ability to filter, warm and humidify air. They work on the principle of capturing heat and moisture exhaled by the patient, which are then returned on inhalation. Furthermore, they will also filter out possible contaminants from both inspired and expired air.

Another 'humidifier' system that is sometimes used is the bubble system, in which the supplemental oxygen is bubbled through sterile water. This is most commonly used with nasal cannulae to alleviate nasal discomfort. However, it has been shown by both Andres et al. (1997) and Campbell et al. (1988) that these systems at flows of less than 5 l/min only distribute water droplets along the narrow bore tubing and therefore do not increase the humidity of the supplemental oxygen, nor do they make any subjective difference to symptoms such as nasal discomfort. Furthermore, they have also been shown to pose an increased infection risk (Cameron et al., 1986). As there is no evidence of clinical benefit and a potential infection risk, the bubble 'humidifier' system should not be used.

Acute oxygen therapy

Oxygen therapy administered during acute illness and in emergency situations needs to be titrated in order to achieve an agreed oxygen saturation, which, apart from in those at risk of hypercapnic respiratory failure (Type II), is usually aimed at achieving a normal or near-normal oxygen saturation. The level of saturation for oxygen titration will depend on the cause of the hypoxaemia, the age of the patient (as there is a natural decline in oxygen saturation with age (Crapo et al., 1999)) and whether the patient is known or is at risk of hypercapnic respiratory failure (Type II). The British Thoracic Society (2008) suggests that for most conditions, the following target saturation ranges can be used as a guide:

- 94–98% for patients aged below 70
- 92–98% for those aged 70 or above
- 88–92% for those at risk of hypercapnic respiratory failure

Oxygen alert cards, which indicate whether a patient has a history of hypercapnic respiratory failure when administered supplemental oxygen during acute exacerbations, have been successful in ensuring that low-flow oxygen delivered via a Venturi mask is used for titration of oxygen therapy, thereby preventing carbon dioxide retention and respiratory acidosis (Durrington et al., 2005; Gooptu et al., 2006). Patients with underlying respiratory disease, such as COPD, who have a documented episode of hypercapnic respiratory failure, should be provided with an oxygen alert card (Figure 3.4) and a 24% or 28% Venturi mask so they can give it to paramedics and/or on arrival to the emergency department. However, in the event of a life-threatening emergency when a diagnosis or previous history is not available then high concentrations of oxygen should be administered immediately (British Thoracic Society, 2008).

Oxygen Alert Card

Name:

I am at risk of carbon dioxide retention (Type II respiratory failure)

My target oxygen saturation during exacerbations is _____%

Please use my _____% Venturi mask

Use compressed air to drive nebuliser (with 2 l/min oxygen via nasal cannula)

Clinical Contact Details:

_____

_____

_____

_____

Name of healthcare professional determining target oxygen saturation:

_____

Signature: _____

Figure 3.4 Oxygen alert card.

Case study 3.1

David, a 69-year-old man, has COPD and is on home oxygen therapy, using 2 l/min via nasal cannulae for 15 hours per day. He has recently had a viral infection, which has resulted in an exacerbation of his COPD with increased expectoration of sputum which is green in colour. He thought it would get better on its on, however, he is becoming more breathless and therefore decides to call his GP. The GP decides to admit him to hospital, so he calls an ambulance. The paramedics assess David's oxygen levels with pulse oximetry. As his saturation level is 84% on air they decide to administer oxygen therapy. They give David 40% oxygen via a Hudson mask, which corrects his oxygen saturation to 96%. On arrival at hospital his arterial blood gases on 40% oxygen are:

PaO_2	12.1 kPa
SaO_2	96%
$PaCO_2$	7.2 kPa
pH	7.35
HCO_3	26

The arterial blood gases demonstrate that David's hypoxaemia has been corrected on the 40% supplemental oxygen; however this high concentration of oxygen has resulted in carbon dioxide retention. It is therefore decided to reduce the supplemental oxygen to 28% via a

Case study 3.1   (Continued)

Venturi mask, which although reducing his SpO_2 to 88%, also reduces his carbon dioxide levels to 5.9 kPa. Reducing the supplemental oxygen prevents carbon dioxide retention, which if left unchecked could lead to respiratory acidosis.

David's COPD exacerbation, which was the cause of deterioration in his blood gases, is treated with antibiotics, corticosteroids, bronchodilators and diuretics. A target oxygen saturation level of 88–92% is stated on the oxygen prescription as there is a documented risk of hypercapnic respiratory failure in response to high concentrations of oxygen. David is discharged after 48 hours, supported by the respiratory hospital at home team. The respiratory nurse, recognising that David has had delayed treatment of his exacerbation, provides education and a self-management plan so that he recognises early signs of exacerbation and can commence treatment earlier in the future. An oxygen alert card is also provided, which indicates that David has a history of hypercapnic respiratory failure when administered supplemental oxygen during acute exacerbations and that the target oxygen saturation is 88–92%. David and his family are informed that they should give this card to anyone administering oxygen to him, such as paramedics and emergency department staff.

Assessment and monitoring

During acute exacerbations, oxygen levels can fluctuate and will alter with deterioration or improvement of the underlying condition, therefore assessment of the overall condition and monitoring of oxygen levels and carbon dioxide levels are vital. The monitoring of patients requiring oxygen therapy during acute illness should include:

- Arterial blood gases
- Oxygen saturation
- Medical emergency early warning scoring system (Subbe et al., 2001).

Arterial blood gases are essential when initiating acute oxygen therapy as it is necessary to establish if there is hypercapnia and if respiratory acidosis is present. This is necessary so that appropriate oxygen titration can be established and the need to initiate non-invasive ventilation can be determined. Furthermore, if the supplemental inspired oxygen levels are increased then arterial blood gases should be repeated within an hour, although they could be taken after only 20 minutes of the change. This will allow carbon dioxide levels on the different percentages of supplemental oxygen to be compared. A raise in carbon dioxide of greater than 0.5 kPa could mean that the additional oxygen is causing carbon dioxide retention, which if not recognised and acted on could result in respiratory acidosis.

Once the target saturation and range of oxygen delivery has been determined to correct hypoxaemia and prevent hypercapnia, pulse oximetry can be used to monitor oxygen levels so that titration against the oxygen prescription can occur. Pulse oximeters have been shown by Jensen et al. (1998) in a meta-analysis to be accurate within 2% in the range of 70–100% SpO_2. They also showed that pulse oximeters may be inaccurate during severe or rapid desaturation, hypotension, hypothermia and low-perfusion states. For this reason the use of a medical emergency early warning scoring system will alert the clinician of deterioration or factors that may cause pulse oximetry to be inaccurate, indicating the need for arterial blood gases to be repeated. Figure 3.5 summarises the guidance for oxygen prescription for acutely breathless patients.

Case study 3.2

Angela is 28 years old and has had asthma since childhood. Her current asthma medication is beclomethasone 400 mcg twice daily via a metered dose inhaler and spacer and salbutamol prn which she usually needs once or twice per day. Recently she has had a 'cold' and has gradu-ally increased the amount of salbutamol use to five times a day. Angela put her worsening of symptoms down to having a 'cold' resulting in her ignoring the worsening of her asthma. She has had a very bad night, and at 4 am cannot breathe and her salbutamol is having very little effect. She is frightened and calls an emergency ambulance. Her oxygen saturation as recorded by the paramedics was 88%, so they started high-flow oxygen using a non-rebreathing mask at 15 l/min which achieved an acceptable target saturation of 96% (target range 94–98%). On arrival in the emergency department 10 minutes later, she has arterial blood gases taken on oxygen:

PaO_2	13.8 kPa
SaO_2	96%
$PaCO_2$	4.8 kPa
pH	7.39
HCO_3	24

The results of the blood gases demonstrated that she was adequately ventilating as there was no carbon dioxide retention. She received nebulised salbutamol driven by 8 litres of oxygen as this ensured that she continued to receive high-flow oxygen so her target oxygen saturation was achieved, which was monitored continuously using pulse oximetry. Her severe asthma was treated in accordance with the British Thoracic Society (BTS)/Scottish Intercollegiate Guidelines Network (SIGN) guidelines. As her condition stabilised following the administration of nebu-lised bronchodilators and oral corticosteroids, her oxygen was reduced to 40% via a 'Hudson' mask as this was sufficient to maintain her oxygen saturations within the target range. Angela was taken off oxygen once her vital signs had returned to normal, although she continued to have oxygen prescribed so that if her oxygen saturations dropped below 94%, it could be recommenced immediately. Angela stayed in hospital for 48 hours, during which time she con-tinued to be monitored and was provided with education about recognition of deterioration. The respiratory nurse specialist also developed an asthma action plan and Angela was asked to make an appointment in 2 weeks' time with her GP or practice nurse.

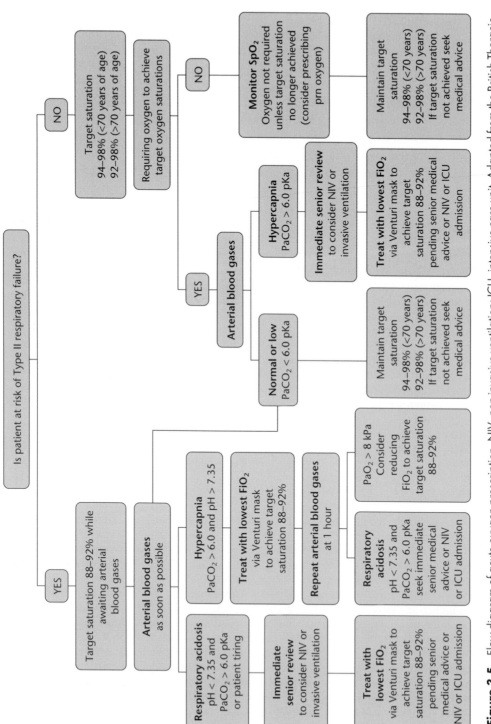

Figure 3.5 Flow diagram of acute oxygen prescription. NIV, non-invasive ventilation; ICU, intensive care unit. Adapted from the British Thoracic Society (2008) guidelines for emergency oxygen use in adult patients.

Is patient at risk of Type II respiratory failure?

YES

Target saturation 88–92% while awaiting arterial blood gases

Arterial blood gases as soon as possible

Respiratory acidosis
pH < 7.35 and
$PaCO_2$ > 6.0 pKa
or patient tiring

Immediate senior review
to consider NIV or invasive ventilation

Treat with lowest FiO_2
via Venturi mask to achieve target saturation 88–92% pending senior medical advice or NIV or ICU admission

Hypercapnia
$PaCO_2$ > 6.0 and pH > 7.35

Treat with lowest FiO_2
via Venturi mask to achieve target saturation 88–92%

Repeat arterial blood gases at 1 hour

Respiratory acidosis
pH < 7.35 and
$PaCO_2$ > 6.0 pKa
seek immediate senior medical advice or NIV or ICU admission

PaO_2 > 8 kPa
Consider reducing FiO_2 to achieve target saturation 88–92%

NO

Target saturation
94–98% (<70 years of age)
92–98% (>70 years of age)

Requiring oxygen to achieve target oxygen saturations

YES

Arterial blood gases

Normal or low
$PaCO_2$ < 6.0 pKa

Maintain target saturation
94–98% (<70 years)
92–98% (>70 years)
If target saturation not achieved seek medical advice

Hypercapnia
$PaCO_2$ > 6.0 pKa

Immediate senior review
to consider NIV or invasive ventilation

Treat with lowest FiO_2
via Venturi mask to achieve target saturation 88–92% pending senior medical advice or NIV or ICU admission

NO

Monitor SpO_2
Oxygen not required unless target saturation no longer achieved (consider prescribing prn oxygen)

Maintain target saturation
94–98% (<70 years)
92–98% (>70 years)
If target saturation not achieved seek medical advice

Home oxygen therapy

There are three categories of home oxygen therapy:

- Long-term oxygen therapy (LTOT)
- Ambulatory oxygen therapy
- Short-burst oxygen therapy

Long-term oxygen therapy

The aim of LTOT is to correct chronic hypoxaemia, which is defined as a PaO_2 of 7.3 kPa or less, and which if left untreated will result in complications of hypoxia which include cor pulmonale, secondary polycythaemia and pulmonary hypertension.

The term LTOT reflects the number of hours that oxygen therapy is used per day rather than how many years oxygen therapy is used for, although once it is commenced, it is likely to be a lifelong treatment. This is based on two randomised controlled trials (Nocturnal Oxygen Therapy Trial, 1980; Medical Research Council, 1981) which demonstrated that if oxygen therapy was used for at least 15 hours per day there was an increase in 5-year survival and an overall improvement in quality of life (Figure 3.6). For this to be achieved it is necessary for

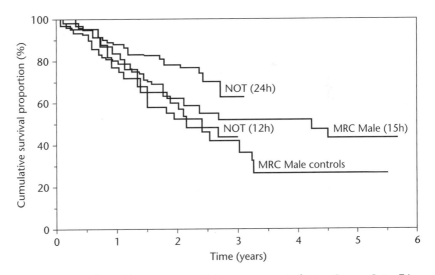

Figure 3.6   Effect of long-term oxygen therapy on survival rates. Source: Petty, T.L., McCoy, R.W. & Doherty, D.E. (2006) Long term oxygen therapy: history, scientific foundations and emerging technologies (6th oxygen consensus conference recommendations). National Lung Health Education Programme. With kind permission of The National Lung Health Education Programme (NLHEP).

the daytime oxygen tension to be kept at or above 8 kPa, which is the equivalent to an oxygen saturation (SpO_2) of 92% or more. As conditions such as COPD progress it is not always possible to maintain oxygen saturation at this level without causing carbon dioxide retention, however, anything less than 90% over a prolonged period will result in secondary complications, such as cor pulmonale. Hence the aim of LTOT is to maintain the oxygen saturation above 90%.

There are several conditions in which LTOT may be indicated:

- COPD
- Cystic fibrosis
- Bronchiectasis
- Interstitial lung disease
- Pulmonary vascular disease
- Primary pulmonary hypertension
- Pulmonary malignancy
- Chronic heart failure

For those with an underlying condition that could result in chronic hypoxaemia screening use of pulse oximetry is advisable. In accordance with guidelines (Royal College of Physicians, 1999; British Thoracic Society, 2006), if the oxygen saturation falls below 92% then a referral should be made for a LTOT assessment, which must include arterial blood gas analysis, so that both oxygen and carbon dioxide levels can be reviewed. During the assessment it is essential that the treatment for the underlying condition is reviewed and optimised. The timing of the assessment also requires consideration as it should take place during a period of clinical stability. Seemungal et al. (2000) demonstrated that it can take up to 6 weeks to recover lung function following an exacerbation of chronic lung disease; therefore if an assessment takes place during this phase, LTOT may be inappropriately prescribed. If, however, during an acute episode there is evidence of hypoxaemia then the British Thoracic Society (2008) recommends that a temporary supply of oxygen is provided for 6 weeks by which time full recovery from the exacerbation will have been achieved. It is recommended in borderline cases that two sets of arterial blood gases during clinical stability should be assessed at least 3 weeks apart as Levi-Valensi et al. (1990) have shown that there can be changes over time. The initial assessment for LTOT should include the following:

- Arterial blood gases on air
- Check for presence of peripheral oedema

- Lung function testing
- Review of medication to ensure optimisation of treatment

If on assessment the PaO_2 is 7.3 kPa or less, repeated arterial blood gases should be undertaken on oxygen. Usually 2 litres oxygen via nasal cannulae is initially used as a starting point for the assessment on oxygen, although this may need to be increased or decreased depending on the results of the arterial blood gases taken while breathing oxygen. Titration should be undertaken to ensure that the PaO_2 is above 8 kPa with no raise in carbon dioxide level compared with when the patient is breathing air.

For patients who have a PaO_2 between 7.3 kPa and 8.0 kPa further assessment may be required to determine if the patient is suitable for oxygen therapy and if indicated, what type of modality is indicated. If there is oedema or pulmonary hypertension and the patient is in a stable phase of their underlying condition, LTOT is indicated. It is also import-ant to ask the patients with this range of arterial blood gases about the effect of exercise on their breathlessness as this may indicate that they are desaturating significantly (SpO_2 < 90%) during activity. If this is suspected, the patient does not need LTOT but will require formal assessment for ambulatory oxygen, to determine if it is the oxygen levels or other factors, such as being physically deconditioned, which are causing the increase in breathlessness on exertion. This will ensure the most appropriate treatment is recommended. For example, the per-son who maintains their SaO_2 above 90% on exercise would benefit from pulmonary rehabilitation rather than oxygen therapy.

Equipment for delivering LTOT

The equipment used to deliver LTOT should be suitable to administer oxygen therapy for at least 15 hours per day, and therefore the use of an oxygen concentrator rather than oxygen cylinders is recommended. An oxygen concentrator (Figure 3.7) runs off a normal household elec-tricity supply, and although it requires to be maintained, it does not require replenishing like an oxygen cylinder would, making it a more convenient and reliable way to supply LTOT. However, there is a chance, although small, that there could be a mechanical breakdown or cessa-tion of the electricity supply, therefore a back-up cylinder should be supplied in case of emergency to anyone using an oxygen concentrator.

An oxygen concentrator provides supplemental oxygen by drawing in room air as a source of the oxygen. Atmospheric air consists of approx-imately 78% nitrogen and 21% oxygen and the aim of the concentrator is

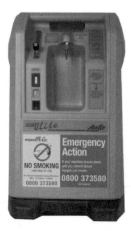

Figure 3.7 Oxygen concentrator. With kind permission from
Air Products Healthcare.

to separate these gases so that an oxygen source is available for use
within the home without the need for constant delivery of cylinders.
This is achieved by use of zeolite which captures nitrogen molecules
from the compressed air drawn into the machine from the atmosphere,
resulting in a continuous supply of oxygen of up to a flow rate of
approximately 5 l/min. The accuracy of delivery depends on the
pressure being maintained. At a flow rate of 2 l/min the concentration
is very accurate at around 95%. However, as the flow rate increases
there can be a reduction in pressure, which reduces the efficiency of the
machine and results in a lower concentration of oxygen. Table 3.2 shows
the range of oxygen concentration at the different flow rates. To overcome this potential reduction and to ensure that the correct flow rate is
prescribed for the patient it is recommended that assessment for LTOT
should be undertaken using an oxygen concentrator rather than cylin-
dered or a piped oxygen supply. Dheda et al. (2004) support this practice as they demonstrated that the oxygen flow required to achieve an
arterial oxygen tension of >8 kPa was significantly greater for an oxygen
concentrator than for wall oxygen, and the difference was most likely
in those with an forced expiratory volume in 1 second (FEV_1) <30% of
predicted.

Table 3.2 Accuracy of oxygen concentrators.

1 l/min	95% ± 3%
2 l/min	95% ± 3%
3 l/min	92% ± 3%
4 l/min	80% ± 3%

The oxygen concentrator is easy to operate and consists of an on/off switch, a flow meter and a pressure alarm. When the machine is first turned on the alarm will sound for a few seconds while the pressure initially builds up to its working pressure. The output is constantly analysed and if the oxygen concentration falls the warning light will flash and the alarm will sound. The most common reason for this occurring is that the filters need changing which is part of the routine maintenance. In addition, the concentrator should be serviced at least every six months in accordance with manufacturer recommendations. The positioning of the oxygen concentrator needs careful consideration in relation to the noise of the machine and therefore a landing, hall or spare room is often chosen. Patients may want to put the concentrator in a cupboard or a wardrobe so it is out of sight, however this should be avoided as there will not be sufficient circulating air.

Oxygen interfaces used with oxygen concentrators

The most common interface used by patients on LTOT is nasal cannulae as this does not impede communication and allows the patient to eat while using oxygen. Furthermore, it is less obvious, which for those patients who are self-conscious about wearing oxygen, can impact on the patient being able to achieve a minimum of 15 hours of oxygen per day. Nasal cannulae are designed to deliver low-flow oxygen, usually 1–4 l/min. Higher flows may cause the nasal passages to become dried out as it is beyond the ability of the cilia within the nose to be able to provide humidification to counteract the dryness of the supplemental oxygen. However, there may be circumstances in which higher flow rates are required, but the impact of the oxygen on the nasal passages needs to be considered because inflammation may result in nose bleeds and pain, which could affect adherence with treatment. It is also important to remember that when the nasal cannula is used in conjunction with an oxygen concentrator, the flow rate accuracy will reduce as the flow rate is increased. Table 3.3 outlines the approximate percentage of oxygen that the various flow rates via nasal cannulae deliver via an oxygen concentrator. In addition, the number of oxygen concentrators required to deliver the different percentages is also indicated as most concentrators can only deliver a maximum of 4 l/min.

Face masks are less likely to be used to deliver LTOT at home as they can be a barrier to communication; also, they need to be removed while the patient is eating or drinking. However, there may be circumstances that warrant a mask being used, for example presence of nasal defect or high flow rates not being tolerated via nasal cannulae. The most

Table 3.3   Approximate percentage of oxygen that the various flows rates via nasal cannulae deliver via an oxygen concentrator.

Per cent	Flow rate	Number of concentrators
24	1 l/min	1
28	2 l/min	1
29.5	3 l/min	1
31	4 l/min	1
33	5 l/min	2
35	6 l/min	2
37.5	7 l/min	2
40	8 l/min	2

Table 3.4   Venturi mask used in connection with oxygen concentrator.

Per cent	Barrel colour	Flow rate	Number of concentrators
24	Blue	2 l/min	1
28	White	2 l/min or 4 l/min	1
31	Orange	6 l/min	2
35	Yellow	8 l/min	2
40	Red	10 l/min	3
60	Green	15 l/min	4

appropriate type of mask is a fixed performance device in the form of a Venturi mask as this will deliver a more accurate concentration of oxygen. When a mask is used it is also advisable to provide the patient with nasal cannulae, so that they can continue to use the oxygen while eating and drinking. Table 3.4 outlines the approximate percentage of oxygen that the various coloured Venturi barrels deliver and what flows rates are used to deliver the required percentage via an oxygen concentrator and the number of oxygen concentrators required to deliver the different percentages is also indicated.

Case study 3.3

Joan is a 72-year-old woman with COPD, who lives with her husband in a two-bedroom maisonette which has a small garden. She has recently been admitted to hospital with an acute exacerbation which was triggered by a viral infection. While in hospital she received 28% oxygen via a Venturi mask, antibiotics, corticosteroids and bronchodilators. She is ready to be discharged and the healthcare team caring for her is wondering if she will require LTOT. Her current arterial blood gases are:

PaO$_2$	7.1 kPa
SaO$_2$	87%
PaCO$_2$	5.1 kPa
pH	7.37
HCO$_3$	25

The arterial blood gases demonstrate that Joan has Type I respiratory failure as her PaO$_2$ is <8.0 kPa, which is equivalent to a SpO$_2$ of approximately <92%. The aim of LTOT is to maintain the PaO$_2$ >7.3 kPa, which is equivalent to a SaO$_2$ of >90%. Based on these results it would appear that Joan would require LTOT, however this may not be so due to these arterial blood gases being taken during an exacerbation of COPD. Seemungal et al., 2000 have demonstrated that it can take up to 6 weeks for lung function, and hence arterial blood gases, to return to a stable state after an exacerbation. Joan had ankle oedema on admission, which was successfully treated with diuretics, suggesting that the hypoxaemia was causing heart failure secondary to respiratory failure (cor pulmonale). This along with her arterial blood gas results indicates that she will require oxygen therapy at home until she recovers from her exacerbation. A decision to order a temporary supply of home oxygen therapy was made and 2 l/min via nasal cannulae was provided to Joan via an oxygen concentrator. A clear explanation of why she needed oxygen at home was given to Joan and her husband, emphasising that this may only be required until she recovered from this exacerbation which can take up to 6 weeks. She was given an outpatient appointment in 6 weeks' when a decision about the need for LTOT would be made. At the 6-week follow-up appointment, Joan had no visible ankle oedema and had no diuretics since she was discharged. She had been using the oxygen overnight and although initially when she was discharged she used it for long periods of the day, she now is using it only overnight. Her arterial blood gases taken during a stable clinical state are:

PaO$_2$	7.9 kPa
SaO$_2$	92%
PaCO$_2$	5.1 kPa
pH	7.37
HCO$_3$	25

The repeated arterial blood gases indicate that Joan does not require LTOT at the moment and this was explained to Joan and her husband. They were also advised that arrangements for the oxygen concentrator to be removed would be made. It was also emphasised that if at a later stage she required home oxygen again, either temporarily or longer term, then this could be easily arranged, but at the present time she has sufficient oxygen in her blood without requiring an additional supply. Joan and her husband were given the opportunity to ask questions so that they understood the reason for the oxygen concentrator being removed.

Case study 3.4

Frank is a 64-year-old man with COPD and lives alone in a first-floor flat. He has had three exacerbations in the past year and when he attends a follow-up appointment it is noted that there has been a decline in his overall lung function (FEV$_1$ 0.9, forced vital capacity (FVC) 1.95). Also, he is complaining of worsening breathlessness, which has affected his ability to go out. An arterialised earlobe gas is taken, and the results are as follows:

Case study 3.4 (Continued)

PaO$_2$	6.9 kPa
SaO$_2$	87%
PaCO$_2$	4.9 kPa
pH	7.38
HCO$_3$	25

Frank had not had an exacerbation of his COPD for the past 2 months and a review of his medication demonstrates that this has been fully optimised. On examination there is peripheral oedema, suggesting that Frank has heart failure which is likely to be secondary to chronic hypoxaemia. His last out-patient blood gases were reviewed, which demonstrated that 4 weeks previously his PaO$_2$ was 7.1 kPa. It was decided that Frank required LTOT, based on the following criteria:

- PaO$_2$ < 7.3 kPa on two occasions at least 3 weeks apart.
- Clinically stable as not had an exacerbation in the past 6 weeks.
- Presence of peripheral oedema.
- FEV$_1$ < 1.0 litres.
- Medical treatment optimal.

The plan is to commence Frank on 2 l/min via nasal cannulae. However, to ensure his hypoxaemia is corrected without carbon dioxide retention, a blood gas is taken on the 2 litres of oxygen. The results are as follows:

PaO$_2$	8.9 kPa
SaO$_2$	94%
PaCO$_2$	4.92 kPa
pH	7.37
HCO$_3$	25

It is clear from the results that 2 litres of oxygen via nasal cannulae is appropriate as the PaO$_2$ is >8.0 kPa and there is no significant change in the PaCO$_2$. To have maximal benefit Frank is informed that he will need to use the LTOT for 15 hours per day. His initial reaction was that this was not possible, however, by planning its use around his life-style and routines, Frank realised that it would be possible to achieve. Frank had already seen the oxygen concentrator as it was used to deliver his oxygen when his blood gases were taken as part of the assessment for LTOT, however, further explanation was provided on how to use the machine, how and when it will be installed, best position for the machine, reimbursement of electricity, maintenance and safety aspects particularly in relation to smoking. The oxygen was ordered and an oxygen concentrator was installed in Frank's flat 3 days later. In addition, a back-up cylinder was provided in case of emergencies such as mechanical breakdown or electricity failure. A follow-up home visit was undertaken by the respiratory nurse 2 weeks later to continue the education and answer questions that Frank had. At that visit the respiratory nurse monitored his SpO$_2$ which was still 94%, checked for peripheral oedema and took the opportunity to discuss self-management of exacerbations. A further visit was planned for 3 months time, but in the meantime Frank was provided with contact numbers of the community respiratory team and home oxygen company.

Ambulatory oxygen therapy

Ambulatory oxygen therapy refers to the provision of oxygen during exercise and activities of daily living for patients who have chronic hypoxaemia or exercise oxygen desaturation (Royal College of Physicians, 1999). The purpose of ambulatory oxygen is to enable the patient to leave the home for a longer period of time, to improve daily activities and quality of life. Ambulatory oxygen has been shown to increase exercise capacity and reduce exertional breathlessness in patients with chronic lung disease (Davidson et al., 1988; Dean et al., 1992; Leach et al., 1992; Eaton et al., 2002). The physiological benefits have been well evaluated, however, despite correction of hypoxaemia and reduction in breathlessness many patients supplied with ambulatory oxygen appear to spend relatively little time outside the home and do not use their equipment on a regular basis (McDonald et al., 1995). Eaton et al. (2002) identified the need to assess more than the physiological measurements which have been traditionally used to determine which patients would benefit from ambulatory oxygen therapy. By using health-related quality of life (HRQOL) measures including validated tools such as the Chronic Respiratory Disease Questionnaire (CRDQ) and the hospital anxiety and depression scale (HAD), they demonstrated significant improvements in HRQOL for patients using ambulatory oxygen over a 12-week period. Despite physiological and quality of life benefits, Eaton et al. (2002) also identified that a substantial proportion of patients declined ambulatory oxygen. It would therefore appear that there are other factors that determine usage of ambulatory oxygen, beyond physiological markers and HRQOL. No studies have determined the long-term effectiveness of ambulatory oxygen – as identified by a Cochrane review conducted in 2002 and updated in 2004, which showed no additional research (Ram & Wedzicha, 2002). It would therefore appear that there are individual factors that may determine if the patient will use the ambulatory oxygen, and which need to be taken into account.

Patients who may be suitable for ambulatory oxygen therapy can be divided into two main categories:

- A PaO_2 of 7.3 kPa or less, or in other words those who are already on LTOT.
- A PaO_2 between 7.3 kPa and 8.0 kPa who desaturate on exercise.

Those already assessed to be appropriate for LTOT are known to meet the criteria for ambulatory oxygen therapy, however there are several factors that need to be taken into account prior to deciding if the patient is going to be supplied with an ambulatory supply of oxygen:

- Do they go out of their home?
- Are they willing to wear nasal cannulae when outside the home?
- When they are outside the home do they use a wheelchair?
- When they are outside the home how long are they mobile or walking for?

Asking these simple questions will determine if further assessment is required. For patients who do not leave the home or clearly state that they are not willing to wear nasal cannulae in public, it would not be appropriate to provide an ambulatory supply of oxygen. Although if circumstances change, then it may be appropriate to reconsider this decision. For example, following a pulmonary rehabilitation programme the patient may physically and emotionally be able to leave the home and to cope better with body image changes of wearing nasal cannulae in public. For those who have limited mobility (i.e. wheelchair or electric scooter) there is no need to undertake any additional assessment as the LTOT assessment will be sufficient. This is because it is known that their PaO_2 at rest will be 7.3 kPa or less (SpO_2 approximately <90%). However, if the patient is willing to use ambulatory oxygen therapy and is mobile outside the home, further assessment is required, so that the flow rate to correct the SpO_2 to above 90% can be determined. This assessment should be undertaken during a phase of stability and should involve either a timed walking test or a shuttle walking test. Figure 3.8 summarises the decision-making process in relation to ambulatory oxygen assessment.

Timed walk test

The timed walk test has been described by McGavin et al. (1976). The patient is asked to walk for either 6 or 12 minutes 'as if late for appointment'. The patient is allowed to rest during the test if they are symptomatic and then restart when symptoms subside. One of the problems encountered with this type of test is that it is not as reproducible as the shuttle walk test as it is difficult to standardise the encouragement during the test. For this reason if serial tests are required, for example in research studies, Guyatt et al. (1984) recommend that 3 practice walks are undertaken, as performance will potentially increase with each walk. Six minutes is usually the choice of timed test as Butland et al.

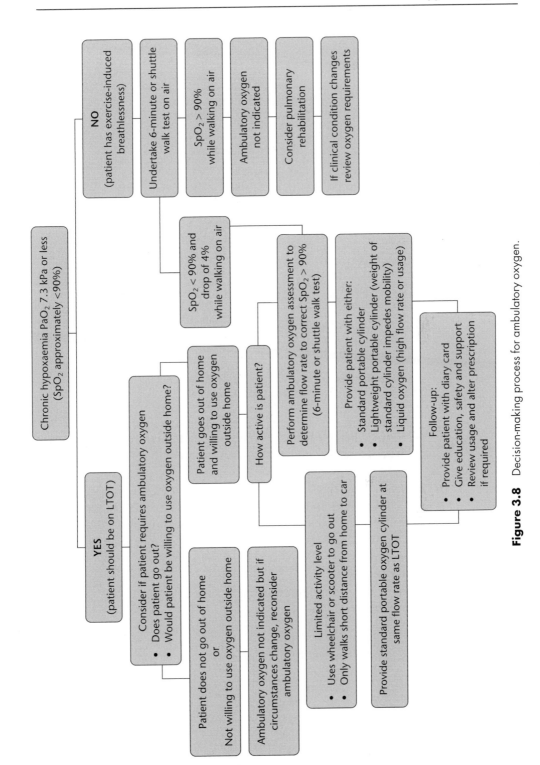

Figure 3.8 Decision-making process for ambulatory oxygen.

Score	Severity
0	No breathlessness at all
0.5	Very very slight (just noticeable)
1	Very slight
2	Slight breathlessness
3	Moderate
4	Somewhat severe
5	Severe breathlessness
6	
7	Very severe breathlessness
8	
9	Very very severe (almost maximum)
10	Maximum

Figure 3.9   Borg score. With kind permission from American Review of Respiratory Medicine.

(1982) showed that the 6- and 12-minute walk tests were comparable for outcomes. The measurements recorded as part of the test are:

- Pre-walk (on air) SpO_2 and heart rate using a pulse oximeter.
- Pre- and post-walk Borg score (Burdon et al., 1982) (Figure 3.9) or visual analogue scale (VAS) for breathlessness (Figure 3.10).
- During walk SpO_2 recording – lowest SpO_2 maintained for at least 30 seconds.
- Distance walked.
- Number of rests and time resting.
- Recovery time.

Please insert a mark along the 10 cm line in relation to the words printed below

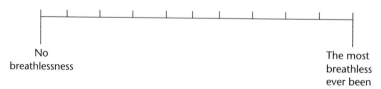

No breathlessness

The most breathless ever been

Figure 3.10   Visual analogue scale (VAS).

Six-minute Walk Test								
Name of patient:				Diagnosis:				
Date of birth:				Date of test:				

On:	At rest	Lowest SpO$_2$/highest HR	At end of test
SpO$_2$			
HR			
BORG		████████	

Distance walked:
Number of rests: Total time resting:
Recovery time:

	20 m	40 m	60 m	80 m	100 m	120 m	140 m	160 m	180 m
SpO$_2$									
HR									

	200 m	220 m	240 m	260 m	280 m	300 m	320 m	340 m	360 m
SpO$_2$									
HR									

	380 m	400 m	420 m	440 m	460 m	480 m	500 m	520 m	540 m
SpO$_2$									
HR									

Figure 3.11 Six-minute walk test results.

It is necessary to record this information at the time of the test and therefore a form should be used so that all required information is captured (Figure 3.11).

Shuttle walk test

The shuttle walk test was developed by Singh et al. (1992) as an incremental, maximal, externally paced test which unlike the 6-minute walk test is not limited by symptoms. This test is reproducible after only one practice walk, which is important when undertaking serial measurements as are often required in research studies. When undertaking assessment for clinical purposes reproducibility may be less important, although it should not be discounted. For patients with restricted mobility due to other underlying conditions, such as rheumatoid arthritis, this test may not be the most suitable as the number of shuttles at the required pace may be difficult to achieve. The 6-minute walk test, where the patient can pace themselves, may be more appropriate as this will replicate what the patient would normally do.

When undertaking the shuttle walk test, the patient walks around two cones which are set 10 metres apart and one shuttle is counted when the patient has walked around the cone and returned to the starting point. The speed at which the patient walks is determined by pre-set bleeps on a tape, which increase every minute. The patient stops walking when they can no longer keep up with the bleeps. At this point it is important to ask what has been the cause for stopping, as often it is presumed that it is breathlessness. In those who lack fitness it may be due to leg fatigue. The measurements recorded as part of the test are:

- Pre-walk (on air) SpO_2 and heart rate using a pulse oximeter.
- Pre- and post-walk Borg score (Figure 3.9) or visual analogue scale (VAS) for breathlessness (Figure 3.10).
- During walk SpO_2 – recording lowest SpO_2 maintained for at least 30 seconds.
- Number of shuttles (distance walked).
- Shuttle walk test level achieved.

For patients who are still able to keep pace with the bleeps until the end of the tape, a modified shuttle walk test (Bradley et al., 2000) may be used as this allows the patients to increase the pace so that they are 'jogging' by the end of the test. This may be suitable for younger patients with a greater level of fitness, such as those with cystic fibrosis. The results of the shuttle walk test need to be recorded during the walk so that the test results are accurate (Figure 3.12).

Once the test is complete the results should be explained to the patient and the outcome of the test summarised so that test and outcome can be communicated to other members of the healthcare team (Figure 3.13).

Equipment to deliver ambulatory oxygen therapy

Once the 6-minute or shuttle walk test has been completed and the patient has recovered, they should be asked about how they felt walking with the oxygen, particularly in relation to the weight of the cylinder, as for some patients the weight of carrying the cylinder may outweigh the

Shuttle Walk Test

Name of patient: Diagnosis:

Date of birth: Date of test:

On:	At rest	Lowest SpO₂/highest HR	At end of test
SpO$_2$			
HR			
BORG		■■■■■■■■■■	

Number of shuttles:

Recovery time: Level achieved:

	Level 1			Level 2			Level 3			
	10 m	20 m	30 m	40 m	50 m	60 m	70 m	80 m	90 m	100 m	110 m	120 m
SpO$_2$												
HR												

	Level 4						Level 5					
	130 m	140 m	150 m	160 m	170 m	180 m	190 m	200 m	210 m	220 m	230 m	240 m	250 m
SpO$_2$												
HR												

	Level 6							
	260 m	270 m	280 m	290 m	300 m	310 m	320 m	330 m
SpO$_2$								
HR								

Figure 3.12   Shuttle walk test results.

benefit of the supplemental oxygen. If this is the case, alternative ways of carrying the cylinder, such as in a shopping trolley or walker should be explored as this may allow the patient to overcome the weight and make the use of ambulatory oxygen more acceptable. The outcome of the walk test should be discussed with the patient and the treatment options explored with them so that an informed decision can be made. Even when physiologically ambulatory oxygen is indicated, the patient may need some time to think about its acceptability.

Ambulatory Oxygen Assessment Outcome	
Patient name:	GP:
Hospital number:	
NHS number:	
Date of birth:	
Patient address:	Consultant:
Phone number:	Lung diagnosis:
Current mobility: Distance Use of aids	Risk factors identified: Angina Yes/No CHD Yes/No Recent MI Yes/No Falls Yes/No Other:
Has patient attended pulmonary rehabilitation: Yes/No Is patient already on long-term oxygen therapy (LTOT) Yes/No	

AMBULATORY ASSESSMENT RESULTS

Type of exercise test:	6-minute walk ☐		Shuttle test ☐		Other (state)			
	Date	O_2 (l/min or %) to correct >90%	SpO_2 at rest	Lowest SpO_2 during test	Walking distance/ No. shuttles	Borg/VAS pre	Borg/VAS post	Usage Hours/day
Assessment on air		■						■
Assessment on oxygen								
Patient able to trigger conserving device Yes/No								
Outcome of ambulatory oxygen assessment:								
Assessment undertaken by:								

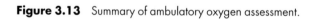

Figure 3.13 Summary of ambulatory oxygen assessment.

Different types of equipment can be used to deliver ambulatory oxygen.

Compressed gas cylinder

Compressed gas cylinder usually come as a standard size weighing 3.2 kg which at 2 l/min will last approximately 3.5 hours; a lightweight option weighing 2.1 kg at 2 l/min lasts approximately 2.5 hours (Figure 3.14). The standard size cylinder is suitable for patients who have limited mobility or have someone or something, such as a scooter or trolley, to carry it. However, for patients who are mobile and can and want to carry their own cylinder, the lightweight option is most suitable.

It is possible to increase the duration of the cylinder by including an oxygen-conserving device (Figure 3.15) which will only deliver oxygen

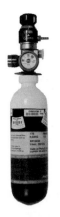

Figure 3.14 Lightweight portable cylinder. With kind permission from Air Products Healthcare.

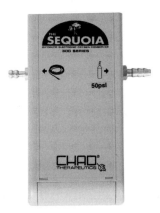

Figure 3.15 Oxygen-conserving device. With kind permission from Air Products Healthcare.

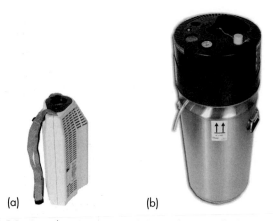

(a)   (b)

Figure 3.16   Liquid oxygen system. (a) Liquid oxygen flask. (b) Liquid oxygen Dewar. With kind permission from Air Products Healthcare.

on inspiration thereby increasing the time the oxygen lasts by approximately three times (e.g. lightweight cylinder at 2 l/min can last for around 7.5 hours). It is triggered by the patient and therefore it is essential that the patient is assessed using it, as mouth breathers or those requiring high flow rates may not be able to sufficiently trigger the device.

Liquid oxygen

Liquid oxygen (Figure 3.16) equipment comprises of two parts, the tank or 'Dewar' and a refillable portable unit which weighs approximately 2.5 kg. The advantage of liquid oxygen is that it lasts longer (2 l/min lasts for 4–5 hours on continuous flow and up to 17 hours on pulse flow, as like the oxygen-conserving devices it delivers the oxygen only on inspiration). The disadvantage is that if it is not used it will evaporate within 2 days, so it is suitable for patients who go out regularly or require high flow rates. Also the patient has to be able to or ask somebody else to refill the portable unit from the Dewar.

Portable concentrator

Portable concentrators (Figure 3.17) work on the same principle as the oxygen concentrators used to deliver LTOT, although they are smaller and are able to run off a battery as well as mains electricity. They are currently quite expensive, although it is anticipated that the cost will come down as they are used more. They are ideal for patients going on holiday, although patients should be assessed on them so that the correct setting can be determined.

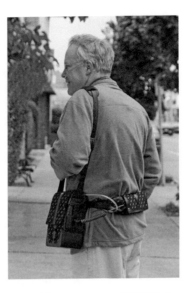

Figure 3.17 Portable concentrator. With kind permission from
Air Products Healthcare.

Case study 3.5

Caroline is 25 years of age and has cystic fibrosis. She has recently been commenced on LTOT at 2 l/min via nasal cannulae. She is using the oxygen for an average of 18 hours per day. Although it was suggested that she should also have ambulatory oxygen, she was asked her opinion about using it. She thought that it would be helpful in getting out of the house and she would be willing to wear nasal cannulae while outside. She was given an appointment for an ambulatory oxygen assessment. A 6-minute walk test was performed and as her SpO_2 was only 86% on air it was not necessary to undertake a walk on air test as she met the criteria for ambulatory oxygen. She then undertook a 6-minute walk test on 2 l/min of oxygen and her results are shown in Table 3.5.

Table 3.5

	O_2 (l/min or %) to correct >90%	SaO_2 at rest	Lowest SaO_2 during test	Walking distance	Borg/VAS	
					Pre	Post
Assessment on oxygen	2 litres	93%	88%	220 m	3	5

Case study 3.5 (Continued)

Table 3.6

	O$_2$ (l/min or %) to correct >90%	SaO$_2$ at rest	Lowest SaO$_2$ during test	Walking distance	Borg/VAS Pre	Post
Assessment on oxygen	4 litres	96%	92%	240 m	3	4

Although Caroline corrected her oxygen levels adequately (SpO$_2$ > 90%) on 2 litres at rest she was desaturating on exercise, resulting in inadequate correction. Therefore following a rest to fully recover from the first walk a second one was undertaken on 4 l/min. The results are shown in Table 3.6.

The 6-minute walk test demonstrated that Caroline corrected her SpO$_2$ on 4 l/min and she was less breathless than when on 2 litres. She was able to trigger the oxygen conserver and the addition of the device did not affect her SpO$_2$. Arterialised blood gases were also checked and there was no carbon dioxide retention noted on either 2 litres or 4 litres of oxygen. The results of the test were discussed with Caroline and she decided that she wanted to have ambulatory oxygen as she felt it would allow her to continue to work as a part-time computer programmer. As she required 4 litres flow rate and because she would be using it for about 4 hours per day it was decided that a liquid oxygen system would be most suitable. A risk assessment was undertaken to ensure that the Dewar could be stored safely in the home and also that Caroline was able to refill her portable unit. Caroline was a non-smoker but she was still advised of the dangers of smoking in case someone visiting her was a smoker. Her liquid oxygen was then ordered and she was advised to have it on 4 l/min when she is walking but to continue on 2 l/min at rest when she uses either the oxygen concentrator or the liquid system. Caroline was asked to complete a simple diary card identifying how much she was going out, using her ambulatory oxygen and type of activity. Caroline had follow-up both at home and at the cystic fibrosis clinic where her diary was reviewed so that any adjustments in her prescription could be made.

Short-burst oxygen

Short-burst oxygen is where oxygen is used for 10–15 minutes at a time via a static source of oxygen. Unlike LTOT and ambulatory oxygen therapy, where there is hypoxaemia either at rest or on exertion, short-burst oxygen is frequently given to patients with normal oxygen levels, although there is little evidence to support this practice. The reason often given for providing patients with short-burst oxygen is to alleviate breathlessness after exercise. Also some patients use a burst of oxygen prior to exertion, such as climbing stairs. It is important that patients with breathlessness on exertion are assessed with a walk test rather than just being provided short-burst oxygen as some patients may be desaturating on exercise and would benefit from ambulatory oxygen.

The latter has been shown to be beneficial if taken during exertion (Lock et al., 1991; Leach et al., 1992). Furthermore, for patients with normal oxygen levels who are experiencing breathlessness on minimal exertion, pulmonary rehabilitation may be a more appropriate treatment option. As there is little evidence to support the use of short-burst oxygen, other treatment options such as breathing exercises and pulmonary rehabilitation should be considered ahead of short-burst oxygen. The guidance from the British Thoracic Society (2006) supports this approach as oxygen should only be prescribed for hypoxaemic patients.

Case study 3.6

Jonathan is 72 years of age and was diagnosed with lung cancer 7 months ago and is now entering the terminal stages of his disease. He lives with his wife in a bungalow and following discussion with the Macmillan Nurse, Jonathan expressed the wish to die at home with support from the Macmillan Nurse, district nursing team and his general practitioner (GP). Although Jonathan does not have hypoxaemia, as he has a SaO_2 of 93%, he does have intermittent breathlessness. His wife requests that her husband is given oxygen as she presumed that lack of oxygen was the cause of his breathlessness. The GP explained that there are other reasons for becoming breathless and that he wanted to arrange for the community respiratory physiotherapist to teach Jonathan breathing control and relaxation techniques as his oxygen SpO_2 did not suggest that oxygen was required. The breathing control and relaxation techniques, and allowing Jonathan to express his concerns about dying, controlled his breathlessness for several weeks. There was then further deterioration and Jonathan was commenced on morphine to control his pain and the increase in breathlessness. This demonstrates the need to fully assess patients who are breathless and supports the wide use of pulse oximetry as part of the initial community assessment. Jonathan died peacefully at home a few days later with his family around him.

Education and support

The benefits of both LTOT and ambulatory oxygen therapy in the chronically hypoxaemic patient are well established, however, the impact on the individual when they are informed they require supplemental oxygen and when they initially start oxygen therapy cannot be underestimated. When introducing the need for home oxygen therapy it is important to emphasise that the aim is to improve quality of life by reducing breathlessness, improving exercise tolerance and reducing frequency of exacerbations.

The following topics should be covered in the education programme:

- Condition requiring LTOT and/or ambulatory oxygen and reason for prescription.
- Explanation of requirements for taking LTOT for at least 15 hours daily and/or discussion of principles of ambulatory oxygen therapy, in relation to individual needs.
- Explanation of the principles of the oxygen concentrator and/or ambulatory oxygen equipment.
- Explanation of home servicing arrangements and electricity reimbursement.
- Discussion of the advantages of using nasal cannulae for oxygen delivery. Some patients may require masks.
- Warning about the dangers of cigarette smoking, gas fires and cookers in the presence of oxygen equipment.
- Installation of oxygen equipment including location and storage.
- Provision of contact telephone numbers for oxygen supplier and healthcare professional (e.g. respiratory nurse).

At follow-up the following should be checked:

- SpO_2 to ensure that hypoxaemia is being corrected ($SpO_2 > 90\%$).
- Oxygen usage with patients and their understanding of importance of adequate compliance.
- Reinforcing that not smoking is essential.
- Assessment of use of ambulatory device if provided.
- Assessment of how patient is coping with oxygen therapy and discuss coping strategies.

In supporting the patient to cope it is necessary to assist the patient to adjust to living with oxygen. Ring & Danielson (1997) identified that patients on LTOT experience:

- **Restriction to time and environment**, which result in feelings of being limited in places to go, length of time able to be out of home (weather, treatment routines), reduced mobility and social isolation.
- **Living at one's own pace**, which requires adaptation to breathlessness and the effect it has on daily life, awareness and acceptance of treatment, and adherence to routine.
- **Put up with LTOT in order to live.**
- **Perception of limitations and managing the situation.**

When a patient commences on home oxygen therapy it is necessary to listen to what the patient's feelings and experiences of being on oxygen are, so that coping strategies can be tailored to the individual, thereby allowing the patient to live with rather than be restricted by the oxygen therapy. As well as individual advice and support the patient may also benefit from pulmonary rehabilitation and also attending a patient support group, such as Breathe Easy (see the British Lung Foundation (BLF) website: www.lunguk.org).

Travelling with oxygen

In order to prevent patients becoming socially isolated it is necessary to ensure that patients on oxygen therapy can travel to either visit friends or family or go on holiday. There are several factors that need to be considered:

- Type of transport when travelling
- Equipment required while away from home
- Length of time away from home

The type of transport when travelling needs considering well in advance of actually going away to ensure that the patient safely arrives at their destination.

Travelling by car

Travelling by car is probably the easiest way of travel as it requires less organisation. However, if oxygen is required to be used or carried in the car a windscreen sticker indicating that oxygen is being carried in the vehicle is recommended, so that in the case of an accident the emergency services are alerted. These stickers are available from the oxygen companies who supply the patient their oxygen. Furthermore, it is advisable that patients inform their car insurance company that they are carrying oxygen in their car. Although this should not increase the cost of the insurance, it will prevent any claim being rejected.

Travelling by train

Travelling by train needs more planning as there are often quite long distances to travel from drop off points to the train. If the patient does not normally have a wheelchair it may be worth considering if it is worth borrowing a wheelchair, for example from the Red Cross, for the period of time the patient is away. Most stations will provide disability assistance, which can be booked in advance, and will ensure the person is escorted to and from the train either in a wheelchair or on a motorised vehicle. Seats should also be booked and if a wheelchair is being used, this needs to be stated at time of booking so that appropriate seats are allocated.

Travelling by aeroplane

Travelling by aeroplane may not be possible for all patients with under-lying respiratory disease as altitude exposure can exacerbate hypox-aemia and those already using LTOT are at particular risk. The cabins of aeroplanes are pressurised to 2438 m (8000 ft) as the international aviation regulations state that this pressure should not be exceeded at a cruising attitude. At this pressure, it is equivalent to breathing 15% oxygen at sea level. The British Thoracic Society (2004) has produced guidelines for predicting in-flight hypoxaemia and the patients requir-ing a fitness to fly assessment (Table 3.7). The initial clinical assessment should include identifying any additional risk factors. According to the British Thoracic Society's guidelines on managing passengers with respiratory disease planning air travel these are:

- $FEV_1 < 50\%$ predicted
- Hypercapnia
- Lung cancer
- Restrictive lung disease involving fibrosis
- Chest wall (kyphoscoliosis) or diseases involving respiratory muscles
- Ventilator support (e.g. non-invasive ventilation)
- Cerebrovascular or cardiac disease
- Within 6 weeks' of discharge for an exacerbation of chronic lung disease

The hypoxic challenge test (Gong et al., 1984) involves breathing 15% inspired oxygen for 15–20 minutes with arterial blood gases being measured before and on completion of the test. Oxygen saturation is also monitored throughout the test for safety. The results of the hypoxic challenge can be divided into three recommendations:

- **No oxygen required** ($PaO_2 > 7.4$ kPa).
- **Borderline** (PaO_2 6.6–7.4 kPa) – a walk test may be helpful as failure to complete the task (in terms of distance or time) or moderate to

Table 3.7 Recommendations for in-flight oxygen.

Screening SaO$_2$ (at sea level)	Assessment recommendations
SaO$_2$ > 95%	No assessment required as SaO$_2$ is normal
SaO$_2$ > 92% with no additional risk factors	No further assessment as in-flight oxygen not required
SaO$_2$ 92–95% with additional risk factors	Hypoxic challenge test required to determine if in-flight oxygen required
SaO$_2$ < 92%	In-flight oxygen required
On long-term oxygen therapy (LTOT)	Increased flow rate of oxygen will be required while at cruising altitude

severe respiratory distress (measured by visual analogue scale) will alert the need for in-flight oxygen.

- **In-flight oxygen required at 2 l/min** (PaO$_2$ 6.6–7.4 kPa).

If a patient requires in-flight oxygen, they should be advised to inform the airline at time of booking so that medical clearance and oxygen will be available during the flight. The airline medical department will require a Medical Information Form (MEDIF) to be completed and this will require the oxygen requirements to be stated. The oxygen on board the aircraft is usually limited to 2 l/min or 4 l/min and this should be considered when the MEDIF is completed by the patient's GP or specialist. It is also important to inform the patient that it is at the discretion of the airline if they charge for the oxygen and also that they may not allow the patient to use their own portable cylinders. To this effect it is therefore advisable to check with the airline prior to booking a holiday so that any additional costs are known in advance.

Oxygen equipment while away from home

As well as organising travelling to the destination it is also necessary for the patient to arrange for oxygen to be available on arrival. In some countries such as the UK, this is available for those already on oxygen in the UK provided it is ordered in advance, ideally 6 weeks prior to travel. However, when travelling outside the country of residence, the patient should be informed that they are likely to be charged for the oxygen. The oxygen companies that supply them their oxygen at home will be able to either organise or provide the patient with a contact within the country they are travelling. Furthermore, the patient should check that the place they are staying is willing to accept the supply of oxygen.

References

American Thoracic Society (2004) COPD guidelines. Available at: www. thoracic.org (accessed 17 May 2008).

Andres, D., Thurston, N., Brant, R., Flemons, W., Fofonoff, D., Ruttimann, A., Sveinson, S. & Neil, C. (1997) Randomized double-blind trial of the effects of humidified compared with nonhumidified low flow oxygen therapy on the symptoms of patients. *Canadian Respiratory Journal*, **4** (2), 76–80.

Bradley, J., Howard, J., Wallace, E. & Elborn, S. (2000) Reliability, repeatability, and sensitivity of the modified shuttle test in adult cystic fibrosis. *Chest*, **117**, 1666–1671.

British Thoracic Society (2004) Managing passengers with respiratory disease planning air travel. Available at: www.brit-thoracic.org.uk/ ClinicalInformation/AirTravel/tabid/92/Default.aspx (accessed 17 May 2008).

British Thoracic Society (2006) Clinical component for the home oxygen service in England and Wales. Available at: http://www.brit-thoracic.org.uk/ Portals/0/Clinical%20Information/Home%20Oxygen%20Service/clinical% 20adultoxygenjan06.pdf

British Thoracic Society (2008) Guideline for emergency oxygen use in adult patients. Available at: www.brit-thoracic.org.uk/ClinicalInformation/ EmergencyOxygen/tabid/219/Default.aspx (accessed 17 May 2008).

Burdon, J.G.W., Juniper, E.F., Killian, K.J., Hargreave, F.E. & Campbell, E.J.M. (1982) The perception of breathlessness in asthma. *American Review of Respiratory Diseases*, **126**, 825–828.

Butland, R.J.A., Pang, J., Gross, E.R., Woodcock, A.A. & Gedes, D.M. (1982) Two, six and twelve minute walking tests in respiratory disease. *British Medical Journal*, **284**, 1607–1608.

Cameron, J.L., Reese, W.A., Tayal, V.S., Clark, R.F., Kelso, D., Gonzalez, E.R., Garnett, A.R. & Ornato, J.P. (1986) Bacterial contamination of ambulance oxygen humidifier water reservoirs: a potential source of pulmonary infection. *Annals of Emergency Medicine*, **15** (11), 1300–1302.

Campbell, E.J., Baker, D. & Crites-Silver, P. (1988) Subjective effects of humidification of oxygen for delivery by nasal cannula. *Chest*, **93**, 289–293.

Cham, G.W., Tan, W.P., Earnest, A. & Soh, C.H. (2002) Clinical predictors of acute respiratory acidosis during exacerbation of asthma and chronic obstructive pulmonary disease. *European Journal of Emergency Medicine*, **9** (3), 225–232.

Crapo, R.O., Jensen, R.L., Hegewald, M. & Tashkin D.P. (1999) Arterial blood gas reference values for sea level and an altitude of 1400 meters. *American Journal of Respiratory Critical Care Medicine*, **160** (5 Pt 1), 1525–1531.

Davidson, A.C., Leach, R., George, R.J. & Geddes, D.M. (1988) Supplemental oxygen and exercise ability in chronic obstructive airways disease. *Thorax*, **43**, 965–971.

Dean, N.C., Brown, J.K., Himelman, R.B., Doherty, J.J., Gold, W.M. & Stulbarg, M.S. (1992) Oxygen may improve dyspnea and endurance in patients with chronic obstructive pulmonary disease and only mild hypoxemia. *American Review of Respiratory Diseases*, **146**, 941–945.

Dheda, K., Lim, K., Ollivere, B., Leftley, J., Lampe, F.C., Salisbury, A., Dilworth, J.P. & Rajakulasingum, R.K. (2004) Assessments for oxygen therapy in COPD: are we under correcting arterial oxygen tensions? *European Respiratory Journal*, **24**: 954–957.

Dripps, R.D. & Comroe, J.H. (1947) The respiratory and circulatory response of normal man to inhalation of 7.6 and 10.4 per cent CO_2. *American Journal of Physiology*, **149**, 43–51.

Durrington, H.J., Flubacher, M., Ramsay, C.F., Howard, L.S.G.E. & Harrison, B.D.W. (2005) Initial oxygen management in patients with an exacerbation of chronic obstructive pulmonary disease. *Quarterly Journal of Medicine*, **98** (7), 499–504.

Eaton, T., Garrett, J.E., Young, P., Fergusson, W., Kolbe, J., Rudkin, S. & Whyte, K. (2002) Ambulatory oxygen improves quality of life of COPD patients: a randomised controlled study. *European Respiratory Journal*, **20**, 306–312.

Georgopolous, D. & Anthonisen, N.R. (1990) Continuous oxygen therapy for the chronically hypoxemic patient. *Annual Review of Medicine*, **41**, 223–230.

Gibson, R.L., Comer, P.B. & Beckman, R.W. (1976) Actual tracheal oxygen concentration with commonly used therapy. *Anesthesiology*, **44**, 71–73.

Gong, H., Tashkin, D.P., Lee, E.Y. & Simmons, M.S. (1984) Hypoxia-altitude simulation test. *American Review of Respiratory Diseases*, **130**, 980–986.

Gooptu, B., Ward, L., Ansari, S.O., Eraut, C.D., Law, D. & Davison, A.G. (2006) Oxygen alert cards and controlled oxygen: preventing emergency admissions at risk of hypercapnic acidosis receiving high inspired oxygen concentrations in ambulances and A&E departments. *Emergency Medicine Journal*, **23**, 636–638.

Guyatt, G.H., Pugsley, S.O., Sullivan, M.J., Thompson, P.J., Berman, L., Jones, N.L., Fallen, E.L. & Taylor, D.W. (1984) Effect of encouragement on walking test performance. *Thorax*, **39**, 818–822.

Hoffman, L.A., Johnson, J.T., Wesmiller, S.W., Sciurba, F.C., Ferson, P.F., Mazzocco, M.C. & Dauber, J.H. (1991) Transtracheal delivery of oxygen: efficacy and safety for long-term continuous therapy. *Annals of Otology, Laryngology and Rhinology*, **100**, 108–115.

Jensen, A.G., Johnson, A. & Sandstedt, S. (1991) Rebreathing during oxygen treatment with face mask. The effect of oxygen flow rates on ventilation. *Acta Anaesthesiologica Scandinavica*, **35** (4), 289–292.

Jensen, L.A., Onyskiw, J.E. & Prasad, N.G. (1998) Meta-analysis of arterial oxygen saturation monitoring by pulse oximetry in adults. *Heart and Lung*, **27** (6), 387–408.

Jones, H.A., Turner, S.L. & Hughes, J.M. (1984) Performance of the large-reservoir oxygen mask (Ventimask). *Lancet*, **i** (8392), 1427–1431.

Kampelmacher, M.J., Deenstra, M., van Kesteren, R.G., Melissant, C.F., Douze, J.M.C. & Lammers, J-W.J. (1997) Transtracheal oxygen therapy: an effective and safe alternative to nasal oxygen administration. *European Respiratory Journal*, **10**, 828–833.

Kory, R.C., Bergmann, J.C., Sweet, R.D. & Smith, J.R. (1962) Comparative evaluation of oxygen therapy techniques. *Journal of the American Medical Association*, **179**, 123–128.

Leach, R.M., Davidson, A.C., Chinn, S., Twort, C.H.C., Cameron, I.R. & Bateman, N.T. (1992) Portable liquid oxygen and exercise ability in severe respiratory disability. *Thorax*, **47**, 781–789.

Levi-Valensi, P., Aubry, P. & Rida, Z. (1990) Nocturnal hypoxaemia and long term oxygen therapy in chronic obstructive pulmonary disease patients with a daytime PaO$_2$ of 60–70 mmHg. *Lung* **168** (Suppl), 770–775.

Lock, A.H., Paul, E.A., Rudd, R.M. & Wedzicha, J.A. (1991) Portable oxygen therapy: assessment and usage. *Respiratory Medicine*, **85**, 407–412.

McDonald, C.F., Blyth, C.M., Lazarus, M.D., Marschner, I. & Barter, C.E. (1995) Exertional oxygen of limited benefit in patients with chronic obstructive pulmonary disease and mild hypoxemia. *American Journal of Respiratory and Critical Care Medicine*, **152**, 1616–1619.

McGavin, C.R., Gupta, S.P. & McHardy, G.J.R. (1976) Twelve minute walking test for assessing disability in chronic bronchitis. *British Medical Journal*, **i**, 822–823.

Medical Research Council (1981) Long term domiciliary oxygen therapy in hypoxemic cor pulmonale complicating chronic bronchitis and emphysema: Report of the Medical Research Council Working Party. *Lancet*, **i**, 681–686.

Mitrouska, I., Tzanakis, N. & Siafakas, N.M. (2006) Oxygen therapy in chronic obstructive pulmonary disease. *European Respiratory Journal*, **38**, 302–312.

Nocturnal Oxygen Therapy Trial Group (1980) Continuous or nocturnal oxygen therapy in hypoxaemic chronic obstructive pulmonary disease: a clinical trial. *Annals of Internal Medicine*, **93**, 391–398.

Plant, P.K., Owen, J.L. & Elliott, M.W. (2000) One year period prevalence study of respiratory acidosis in acute exacerbations of COPD: implications for the provision of non-invasive ventilation and oxygen administration. *Thorax*, **55** (7), 550–554.

Ram, F.S. & Wedzicha, J.A. (2002) Ambulatory oxygen for chronic obstructive pulmonary disease. *Cochrane Database of Systematic Reviews*, **2**: CD000238.

Refsum, H.E. (1963) Relationship between state of consciousness and arterial hypoxaemia and hypercapnia in patients with pulmonary insufficiency, breathing air. *Clinical Science*, **25**, 361.

Ring, L. & Danielson, E. (1997) Patients' experience of long term oxygen. *Journal of Advanced Nursing*, **26** (2), 337–344.

Royal College of Physicians (1999) *Domiciliary Oxygen Therapy Services. Clinical Guidelines and Advice for Prescribers*. A report of the Royal College of Physicians, London.

Rudolph, M., Banks, R.A. & Semple, S.J. (1977) Hypercapnia during oxygen therapy in acute exacerbations of chronic respiratory failure. *Lancet*, **ii**, 483–486.

Seemungal, T.R., Donaldson, G.C., Bhowmik, A., Jeffries, D.J. & Wedzicha, J.A. (2000) Time course and recovery of exacerbations in patients with chronic obstructive pulmonary disease. *American Journal of Respiratory Critical Care Medicine*, **161** (5), 1608–1613.

Singh, S.J., Morgan, M.D.L., Scott, S., Walters, D. & Hardman, A.E. (1992) Development of a shuttle walking test of disability in patients with chronic airways obstruction. *Thorax*, **47**, 1019–1024.

Subbe, C.P., Kruger, M., Rutherford, P. & Gemmel, L. (2001) Validation of a modified Early Warning Score in medical admissions. *Quarterly Journal of Medicine*, **94** (10), 521–526.

Waldau, T., Larsen, V.H. & Bonde, J. (1998) Evaluation of five oxygen delivery devices in spontaneously breathing subjects by oxygraphy. *Anaesthesia*, **53** (3), 256–263.

Chapter 4
NON-INVASIVE VENTILATION

Non-invasive ventilation (NIV) involves the use of a nasal or face mask to supply ventilatory support, therefore avoiding the use of an endotracheal tube (National Institute for Clinical Excellence (NICE), 2004). It may also be referred to as non-invasive positive pressure ventilation (NIPPV).

NIV has many advantages over intubation and ventilation, which can carry high levels of mortality particularly in a chronic respiratory disease group such as chronic obstructive pulmonary disease (COPD) (Seneff et al., 1995). Originally developed from early studies using nasal masks in the treatment of nocturnal hypoventilation in neuromuscular disease (Kerby et al., 1987; Ellis et al., 1988), it is now a recognised intervention in the treatment of acute hypercapnic respiratory failure due to exacerbations of COPD (Evans, 2001; British Thoracic Society (BTS) Standards of Care Committee, 2002), in weaning in COPD, in immuno-compromised patients, in post-operative respiratory failure and in cystic fibrosis (Hodson et al., 1991). It is also used for the treatment of chronic hypercapnic respiratory failure in patients with neuromuscular diseases such as Duchenne's muscular dystrophy, myotonic dystrophy (Leger et al., 1994; Simonds et al., 1998), motor neurone disease (Polkey et al., 1999), chest wall disease such as thoracoplasty and kyphoscoliosis (Kerby et al., 1987; Ellis et al., 1988) and in the treatment of selected patients with COPD (Meecham-Jones et al., 1995). This treatment is used in conjunction with conventional or standard treatments which may include oxygen therapy, diuretics, antibiotics, respiratory stimulants and steroids (NICE, 2004).

Indications: acute use (Box 4.1)

Chronic obstructive pulmonary disease

The BTS (2002) guideline 'Non-invasive ventilation in acute respiratory failure' sets out the standards of care for patients receiving NIV and states that NIV has been shown to be effective in the treatment of acute Type II hypercapnic respiratory failure, particularly in COPD. There is now strong evidence supporting the use of NIV in the management of acute exacerbations of COPD (NICE, 2004). COPD is characterised by exacerbation of respiratory failure and between a fifth and a third of all patients admitted to hospital as a result of hypercapnic respiratory failure due to COPD will die despite the use of intubation and ventilation (Bott et al., 1993; Ambrosino et al., 1995; Brochard et al., 1995). Mortality rates have been reported to rise to 59% where patients are admitted to intensive care for intubation as a result of hypercapnic respiratory failure (Seneff et al., 1995).

A Cochrane review of 14 randomised controlled trials concluded that patients with COPD who fitted the criteria should be offered NIV (Ram et al., 2003). This is an important step forward in gaining acceptance of NIV as a form of treatment for these patients. Although the costs of treating this group are high (estimated to be approximately £800 million in the UK in 2002/3 (Respiratory Alliance, 2003); 30 000 deaths per year (1999)), patients with COPD have tended to be a largely undertreated group and NIV services nationally tend to be patchy in provision. In 1997, only 48% of hospitals in the UK offered NIV as a service (BTS Standards of Care Committee, 2002).

The BTS guideline (2002) recommends that NIV should be considered for patients with an acute exacerbation of COPD in whom respiratory acidosis (pH < 7.35) persists despite optimal medical management including oxygen therapy. Studies identified that significant changes in pH, PaO_2 and $PaCO_2$ could be achieved within 1 hour of treatment with NIV (Bott

---

Box 4.1 Conditions for use of NIV.

- Chest wall deformity (e.g. kyphoscoliosis, thoracoplasty)
- Neuromuscular diseases (e.g. muscular dystrophy, motor neurone disease)
- Chronic obstructive pulmonary disease (COPD)
- Obstructive sleep apnoea/hypopnoea syndrome
- Obesity hypoventilation syndrome
- Cystic fibrosis
- Bronchiectasis

et al., 1993; Brochard et al., 1995; Kramer et al., 1995). This is an important finding in terms of the practical application of NIV in the clinical setting.

A study of predictors of success for NIV in patients with acute respiratory failure due to COPD found that unsuccessful episodes of treatment were associated with a severely deranged baseline pH and $PaCO_2$, a low body mass index, the presence of pneumonia, a severe level of neurological deterioration and an inability to comply with ventilation (Ambrosino et al., 1995). In addition, copious respiratory secretions, poor nutritional status and the edentulous state have been associated with poor outcomes with NIV (BTS Standards of Care Committee, 2002). Although it is not possible to predict which patients will have a successful outcome with NIV, it is more likely to occur where patients adapt well to its use and where a good fit of the interface is achieved. In addition, where patients have a less severe physiological derangement together with rapid changes in respiratory rate and pH in response to NIV, improvements in patient outcomes are more likely.

Evidence from studies performed with patients with COPD in the intensive care unit (ICU) show that NIV is feasible and reduces the rate of tracheal intubation: Kramer et al. (1995) found a reduced intubation rate but no change in mortality while Celikel et al. (1998) showed a rapid improvement in physiological parameters but no change in intubation or mortality rates. Studies have also reported the successful use of NIV in the ward setting with varying results. Bott et al. (1993) demonstrated a significant survival benefit in those treated with NIV in the ward setting when patients unable to tolerate NIV were excluded. Barbé et al. (1996) showed little difference between the two groups, but they included patients with small deviations in acidosis who were likely to improve with standard therapy. Plant et al. (2000) demonstrated a reduction in the need for intubation (determined by the identification of treatment failure criteria) from 27% to 15% when using NIV in the ward setting by the use of a simple protocol by the usual ward staff. In addition in-hospital mortality was reduced from 20% to 10%.

Box 4.2 summarises the use of NIV in acute exacerbations of COPD.

Box 4.2   Summary of the use of NIV in acute exacerbations of COPD.

- Decrease in mortality
- Decreased need for intubation
- Improvement in pH and respiratory rate in the first hour of treatment
- Fewer complications (principally ventilator associated pneumonia)
- Shorter duration of hospital stay

Case study 4.1 Use of NIV in acute exacerbation of COPD

Martha is a 74-year-old woman who has COPD and is on long-term oxygen therapy (LTOT) at home. She has been admitted with an acute exacerbation of her COPD and has severe emphysematous lungs. She is to start on antibiotics, corticosteroids, bronchodilators and diuretics to optimise her treatment of her COPD. Despite this, her arterial blood gases on admission on 28% O_2 via Venturi mask were:

pH	7.27
PaO_2	6.2 kPa
SaO_2	83%
$PaCO_2$	10.2 kPa
HCO_3	27

These results demonstrate that Martha is in Type II respiratory failure with uncompensated respiratory acidosis. She was reviewed by the multi-disciplinary team and a management plan agreed, including NIV, resuscitation status and medication. NIV was set up with the following parameters:

Inspiratory positive airway pressure (IPAP): 14
Expiratory positive airway pressure (EPAP): 4
BPM: 10
2 litres O_2

One hour after starting NIV, her arterial blood gases on NIV were:

pH	7.28
PaO_2	11.0 kPa
SaO_2	95%
$PaCO_2$	9.9 kPa
HCO_3	27

To optimise further use of NIV, entrained oxygen was reduced to 1 l/min, as this could be preventing her $PaCO_2$ being reduced. In addition the IPAP was increased to 16, thereby increasing ventilation, as the pH had not changed significantly.

Blood gases were taken an hour after the changes were made, and showed continued improvement. Monitoring of vital signs continued and arterial gases were repeated at 4 hours. After the first 12 hours, Martha was able to have periods off the NIV and a plan of weaning was instituted.

Use of non-invasive ventilation in intensive care units

As well as aiding the avoidance of endotracheal intubation, NIV has been successfully used in weaning from intubation patients who have Type II respiratory failure, resulting in:

- Improvement in arterial blood gases during weaning
- Reduced length of time spent on ventilator
- Reduced incidence of ventilator associated pneumonia
- Reduced hospital stay

Udwadia et al. (1992) and Restrick et al. (1993) demonstrated this in heterogeneous groups of patients which included those with chest wall diseases, neuromuscular diseases and post-operative complications. Udwadia et al. (1992) found the length of time spent on the ventilator was reduced, resulting in a reduced length of hospital stay while Restrick et al. (1993) found significant improvements in both PaO_2 and $PaCO_2$ when NIV was used in weaning from full ventilation. Nava et al. (1998) studied COPD patients randomised to receive standard weaning (pressure support via an endotracheal tube) or extubation followed by NIV and showed significant decreases in time spent receiving mechanical ventilation, increase in the percentage of successfully weaned patients, improvements in survival at 3 months and reduction in incidence of ventilator-associated pneumonia. In a similar study, Girault et al. (1999) found that patients using NIV could be extubated earlier but there was no difference in the number of patients who could be weaned, the time spent in ICU or survival at 3 months. Antonelli et al. (1998) found that those having invasive ventilation had more complications and more had pneumonia or sinusitis related to the endotracheal tube. In addition, patients in the NIV group had shorter length of stays in ICU and shorter periods of ventilation.

The BTS guideline (2002) recommends the use of NIV where conventional weaning strategies have failed.

Chest wall deformity and neuromuscular disease

The use of NIV in the treatment of long-term chronic respiratory failure due to chest wall deformities such as thoracoplasty and kyphoscoliosis, and neuromuscular diseases such as Duchenne's muscular dystrophy, and myotonic dystrophy is now well documented. NIV is therefore recommended as the treatment of choice where acute ventilatory failure occurs in these patient groups (BTS Standards of Care Committee, 2002). Evidence from both the UK (Simonds & Elliott, 1995) and France (Leger et al., 1994) demonstrates long-term survival benefits with home NIV for these patients, a point which will be returned to later in the chapter.

Case study 4.2   Chest wall disease

Angela is 76 years old and is a known patient with kyphoscoliosis secondary to polio at the age of 7. She worked as a secretary and 20 years ago, presented with respiratory failure and the following observations: forced expiratory volume in 1 second (FEV_1) 0.9 litres, FVC 1.1 litres; PaO_2 6.5 kPa, $PaCO_2$ 8.2 kPa and signs of cor pulmonale. At that time, on supplemental oxygen, her arterial blood gases were:

pH	7.25
PaO_2	10.5 kPa
SaO_2	94%
$PaCO_2$	11.0 kPa
HCO_3	31

She was intubated and ventilated, and a tracheostomy performed. She was transferred to a specialist chest hospital for NIV and weaned from IPPV, resulting in the removal of the tracheostomy. Her arterial blood gases on NIV with a volume cycled ventilator were:

pH	7.36
PaO_2	9.1 kPa
SaO_2	93%
$PaCO_2$	6.03 kPa
HCO_3	26

She had regular follow up in a specialist respiratory clinic and went back to work and looking after her elderly mother. Her blood gases remained stable and her ventilator subsequently changed to pressure support. Thereafter she had no hospital admissions due to respiratory failure and only one with chest pain and possible angina. Her arterial blood gases 20 years on are PaO_2 9.3 kPa and $PaCO_2$ 6.4 kPa. This case illustrates the importance of early recognition of respiratory failure especially in patients with restrictive disorders as this group often has normal daytime gases but abnormal overnight gases, illustrating the need for including sleep study in the assessment.

Respiratory failure due to obstructive sleep apnoea/hypopnoea syndrome

The use of continuous positive airway pressure (CPAP), powered by electricity and delivering a pre-set pressure via a nasal mask, has been demonstrated to be an effective treatment for obstructive sleep apnoea/hypopnoea syndrome (OSAHS) (Sullivan et al., 1981) (more detail about the use of CPAP can be found in Chapter 5). However, in the most severe cases, patients with OSAHS develop Type II respiratory failure as a sequela of their condition. In these cases, the use of NIV has been demonstrated to be beneficial (Bott et al., 1991), with the BTS guidelines (2002) recommending the use of bi-level positive pressure.

Case study 4.3   NIV for obesity/hypoventilation syndrome

Martin is a 38-year-old patient with obesity/hypoventilation syndrome. He has a body mass index of 49 kg/m^2 and weighs over 160 kg. He had a sleep study 6 months ago, which showed his condition has been successfully managed with home CPAP up to this point. He gets short of breath on minimal exertion and stopped working recently. His arterial blood gases on room air are usually:

pH	7.34
PaCO$_2$	6.0
PaO$_2$	8.1

His usual CPAP setting is 8.00 cmH$_2$O.
He was admitted to hospital with worsening arterial blood gases on room air:

pH	7.30
PaCO$_2$	8.6
PaO$_2$	4.6

This indicates that Martin's condition is no longer being managed within acceptable limits and that he is now in Type II respiratory failure. He is at major risk from intubation as mortality would be greatly increased by his weight so NIV is a useful adjunct to treatment which can be used to re-set Martin's arterial blood gases while he is an inpatient and may also be considered, after assessment, for use in the long term at home.

Cystic fibrosis and bronchiectasis

There is insufficient evidence to recommend the use of NIV routinely for the treatment of cystic fibrosis and bronchiectasis unless there is a clear indication that there is a reversible element to the acute exacerbation. It is thought that the presence of sputum causes a physiological obstruction, leading to poor outcomes with ventilation. In addition, there are data showing that of all the groups receiving long-term non-invasive ventilation, those with bronchiectasis do least well with a survival rate of 20% at 5 years (Simonds & Elliott, 1995). However, there is evidence to support the use of NIV in providing a successful bridge to transplantation where this is appropriate (Hodson et al., 1991). In practice, a trial of NIV may be offered where both subjective and objective benefits for the patient can be identified, on the basis that it may be withdrawn at the point when it no longer provides benefit, following discussions with the patient and the multi-disciplinary team.

Cardiogenic pulmonary oedema

NIV has been used for the treatment of cardiogenic pulmonary oedema, however results have been conflicting. Masip et al. (2000) reported quicker improvements with NIV when compared to oxygen therapy in patients with acute cardiogenic pulmonary oedema whilst Sharon et al. (2000) reported better outcomes with nitrate infusions compared to treatment with NIV. The use of high-flow CPAP for the treatment of cardiogenic pulmonary oedema, where hypoxia persists despite maximal therapy, is well documented (Pang et al., 1998) and is preferred over NIV in this group (BTS Standards of Care Committee, 2002).

Other conditions

NIV has been used in a variety of other conditions such as pneumonia, acute respiratory distress syndrome, post-operative and post-transplantation respiratory failure, and has resulted in reduced intubation levels, ICU length of stay and mortality. However, there is relatively weak evidence to support the use of NIV to treat these conditions and therefore it is not routinely used for these groups. The recommendation is that those patients who may then go on to intubation and ventilation should receive a trial of NIV in the ICU setting (BTS Standards of Care Committee, 2002). Box 4.3 summarises the indications for acute use of NIV.

Box 4.3 Summary of the indications for the acute use of NIV.

- Acute exacerbation of chronic obstructive pulmonary disease (COPD) pH < 7.35
- Facilitation in weaning in COPD
- Acute-on-chronic hypercapnia respiratory failure due to chest wall deformity or neuromuscular disease
- Decompensated obstructive sleep apnoea (patients should receive bi-level pressure support)
- Cystic fibrosis and bronchiectasis patients with a pH of <7.35 (excessive secretions may limit the degree of effectiveness)
- Acute cardiogenic pulmonary oedema in whom CPAP has been ineffective

Economic indications

There is a move to reduce the number of acute admissions to hospital, however, patients with hypercapnic respiratory failure will always require acute care. Chu et al. (2004) followed 110 patients with acute hypercapnic respiratory failure for one year after they had received NIV acutely in a high dependency unit. One year after discharge, 80% had been readmitted, 63% had another life-threatening event and 49% had died. The authors concluded that urgent work is required to reduce re-admissions and life-threatening episodes in this group of patients. There is a potential for cost savings through reducing length of stay and the number of acute admissions. NIV has been shown to achieve this by Tuggey et al. (2003) in a study of 13 patients with recurrent exacerbations of COPD that analysed the costs and consequences of the use of home NIV. Tuggey et al. (2003) found that the use of home NIV resulted in a saving of £8254 per patient per year. In addition, they identified a reduced length of hospital stay from a mean of 78 to 25 days with attendant reduction in costs. The mean number of admissions fell from 5 to 2 and ICU days fell from a total of 25 to 4.

Indications: long-term use

Chest wall disorders and neuromuscular diseases

The use of long-term home NIV in the treatment of chest wall disorders and neuromuscular diseases has been shown to be effective (Kerby et al., 1987; Ellis et al., 1988). In the home setting, NIV is recommended for use nocturnally in patients with neuromuscular diseases and chest wall disorders and has been shown by Sivasothy et al. (1998), Consensus Conference Report (1999) and Turkington & Elliott (2000) to improve:

- Mortality
- Daytime arterial blood gases
- Quality of sleep

Leger et al. (1994) studied 276 patients in France using nocturnal NIV over a 2-year period. Patients had diagnoses including chest wall disorders, neuromuscular diseases and thoracoplasty resulting from sequelae of tuberculosis. Significant improvements were found in arterial blood gases and reduction in need for hospitalisation once NIV had been commenced in patients with kyphoscoliosis and thoracoplasty. In addition, these patients demonstrated improvements in sleep and activities of daily living. At two years, 80% of the kyphoscoliosis group and 76% of the thoracoplasty group remained on NIV compared with 56% of patients with Duchenne's muscular dystrophy. These findings were corroborated by Simonds & Elliott (1995) in the UK who studied a similar group of patients using NIV over a 5-year period. This study found that the 5-year actuarial probability of continuing NIV in patients with previous polio, post-tuberculous lung disease, neuromuscular disorders and scoliosis was 100%, 94%, 81% and 79%, respectively. This compared more favourably with figures obtained for patients with COPD and bronchiectasis, whose probability of continuing NIV was 43% and 20%, respectively. It is therefore recommended as an early intervention in the long-term treatment for patients with kyphoscoliosis and thoracoplasty.

The clinical indicators for the long-term use of NIV in the treatment of restrictive lung disorders as identified by the Consensus Conference Report (1999) are: symptoms including fatigue, dyspnoea, morning headache and one of the following:

- $PaCO_2 > 6$ kPa.
- Nocturnal desaturation of <88% for 5 consecutive minutes.
- In progressive neuromuscular disease, maximal inspiratory pressure of <60 cmH_2O or a forced vital capacity (FVC) <50% predicted.

Nocturnal hypoventilation

Some patients with restrictive disorders, such as kyphoscoliosis, thoracoplasty and neuromuscular diseases, will have normal daytime arterial blood gases, but they may develop symptoms of Type II respiratory failure overnight due to nocturnal hypoventilation. The clinical indicators for the long-term use of NIV in the treatment of nocturnal hypoventilation as identified by the Consensus Conference Report (1999) are:

- Polysomnograph for the diagnosis of sleep apnoea, not responsive to CPAP
- Indications for the use of NIV
- Central sleep apnoea
- Other forms of nocturnal hypoventilation

Chronic obstructive pulmonary disease

Patients with severe COPD requiring long-term home NIV need to be carefully selected (Simonds & Elliott, 1995). These patients need assessment prior to selection to ensure that the treatment is beneficial in terms of improvements in overnight blood gas analysis. Meecham-Jones et al. (1995) demonstrated improvements in arterial blood gases, improved quality of life and improved sleep in patients with stable COPD using NIV at home compared to the use of oxygen alone. It was recommended that patients with COPD should show correction of arterial blood gases overnight using NIV before this is prescribed for home use (Meecham-Jones et al., 1995).

More recently, Clini et al. (2002) studied 90 stable COPD patients on either LTOT or LTOT plus NIV over 2 years and demonstrated improved quality of life, improved arterial blood gases, decreased dyspnoea and decreased exacerbations. In addition, hospital admissions decreased by 45% in the home NIV group compared with those patients using LTOT alone, who had an increase in hospital admissions of 27% over the two years. Length of admission to the intensive care unit fell in both groups, decreasing by 75% in the group using both LTOT and NIV and by 20% in the group using LTOT alone. Survival in each group was similar. However, Casanova et al. (2000) found that although at 3 months patients with severe COPD using NIV at home had a decreased number of hospital admissions, this did not continue longer term, as at 6 months there was no difference between patients using either LTOT and NIV or LTOT alone. In addition, other outcomes considered in this trial were rate of acute admission, intubations, and mortality, dyspnoea and neuropsychological function at 3, 6 and 12 months. They found that the only additional differences between the two groups were in dyspnoea score and psychomotor co-ordination at 6 months.

The clinical indicators for the use of NIV in the long-term treatment of COPD as identified by the Consensus Conference Report (1999) are: symptoms including fatigue, dyspnoea, morning headache and one of the following:

- $PaCO_2$ of >7.3 kPa (check).
- ± nocturnal desaturation <88% for 5 consecutive minutes on oxygen therapy of 2 litres or greater.
- $PaCO_2$ of 6.7–7.2 kPa and recurrent hospitalisations due to hypercapnic respiratory failure.

Cystic fibrosis and bronchiectasis

In cystic fibrosis and bronchiectasis there is limited evidence to support the use of long-term NIV. Piper et al. (1992) described its use in 4 patients with cystic fibrosis who were hypercapnic and were discharged home with NIV. These patients showed improvements in both $PaCO_2$ and sleep. Gozal (1997) described its use at home in 6 patients with cystic fibrosis who showed improvements in $PaCO_2$ and PaO_2 with overnight use, with no change in sleep architecture. Simonds & Elliott (1995) demonstrated that patients in the high-volume sputum-producing categories, in this case bronchiectasis, faired the least well out of all long-term users of NIV, with a 5-year probability of continuing on NIV of less than 20%. While care should be taken in extrapolating results from one group to another, nevertheless these poor outcomes should be considered when decisions are made about putting high-volume sputum-producers, such as the cystic fibrosis group, on long-term ventilation. Clear evidence of benefit to the patient should be identified before commencing this group on long-term NIV.

Patterns of use of home non-invasive ventilation

The pattern of use of home mechanical ventilation in Europe was studied by Lloyd-Owen et al. (2005) who identified a total of 27 118 home NIV users. A total of 483 centres treating home NIV users were asked to identify the cause of respiratory failure. Three disease categories were identified:

- Lung and airways disease (including COPD, bronchiectasis, cystic fibrosis).
- Thoracic cage abnormalities (including kyphoscoliosis, thoracoplasty, obesity hypoventilation syndrome).
- Neuromuscular diseases (including muscular dystrophy, motor neurone disease, spinal cord damage and phrenic nerve palsy).

Patients with lung diseases usually used home NIV for less than a year, while patients with thoracic cage disorders usually used home NIV for 6–10 years and patients with neuromuscular diseases more than 6 years. In the survey 34% of home NIV users in Europe had a diagnosis of lung disease, the majority of whom would have had COPD, indicating the widespread use of NIV for the treatment of patients with this disease.

Case study 4.4   Long-term use in COPD

Harry is a 72-year-old man with COPD. At the age of 48, he presented with shortness of breath, airflow obstruction (FEV_1 45% predicted), hypoxaemia (PaO_2 6.61 kPa; $PaCO_2$ 6.86 kPa) and secondary polycythaemia. He had been a cigarette smoker since the age of 14. At that time, he was treated with bronchodilators, oral steroids, venesection for his polycythaemia and his FEV_1 improved to 60% predicted and PaO_2 to 9.1 kPa. He had continued to smoke and he presented with worsening FEV_1 and was started on home oxygen at the time. Twelve years after diagnosis, his FEV_1 had dropped to 37% predicted and his blood gases on air were:

pH	7.39
PaO_2	6.38 kPa
SaO_2	83%
$PaCO_2$	8.07 kPa
HCO_3	29

Harry had had repeated GP visits and hospital admissions. Due to increasing number of hospital admissions he was started on home NIV via BiPAP and oxygen at 2 l/min. Initially he had some problems with compliance and needed a short hospital admission to help with this. This required co-ordination of his care to ensure that all healthcare staff looking after Harry were educated and Harry had a contact healthcare professional who could answer specific queries in relation to his NIV. Two years later his arterial blood gases were:

pH	7.36
PaO_2	8.44 kPa
SaO_2	93%
$PaCO_2$	6.77 kPa
HCO_3	26

Harry was on maximal inhaled therapy for the treatment of his COPD and this, in combination with NIV, resulted in no hospital admissions for 18 months. Although there has been some deterioration in the progression of his COPD, the addition of NIV with entrained oxygen has maintained his PaO_2 at 8.62 kPa and $PaCO_2$ at 6.74 kPa. He remains stable and compliant with NIV and has regular follow up with his specialist respiratory team and supported by regular visits from the community matron, who has organised appropriate social support.

Indications: palliation

The use of NIV in the palliation of terminal symptoms has been documented in the treatment of some chronic diseases including cystic fibrosis (CF) and progressive neuromuscular diseases such as Duchenne's muscular dystrophy and motor neurone disease.

Cystic fibrosis

In cystic fibrosis, NIV has been used to palliate symptoms, such as breathlessness, and as a bridge to transplantation. Patients should be enabled to make choices about how and when they use NIV in the terminal stages of their disease with adequate support for alternative palliative care measures.

The successful use of NIV as a bridge to transplantation in patients with cystic fibrosis is described by Hodson et al. (1991), Hill et al. (1998) and Madden et al. (2002), who concluded that the indications for NIV in this group was as a bridge to transplantation. Hodson et al. (1991) used NIV in six patients awaiting transplantation for between 3 and 17 days; two patients died while on the transplant list while four went on to have successful transplants. Hill et al. (1998) demonstrated successful use of NIV in 10 patients with cystic fibrosis for between 1 and 15 months with improvements in FVC, $PaCO_2$, and inpatient stay at 3 months and subjective improvements in headache and quality of sleep. In this group, three patients went on to transplantation, four died and at the end of the study, three continued to remain on the transplant list. Madden et al. (2002) describes the outcome of a larger group of cystic fibrosis patients using NIV, who were ascribed to one of three groups according to their transplant status: 65 patients were waiting for transplantation, of whom 23 received a transplant and of whom 12 lived. Twenty-five patients were assessed for transplant, five of whom received a transplant, and of whom four lived. There were 23 patients in the group which was not going for transplantation – 20 of whom died. In each group, arterial hypoxaemia was corrected by NIV but hypercapnia remained uncorrected.

Neuromuscular diseases

The use of NIV in progressing neuromuscular diseases such as Duchenne's muscular dystrophy and motor neurone disease has been shown to be beneficial in controlling symptoms caused by severe hypercapnic respiratory failure. Polkey et al. (1999) recommend early discussions about the use of NIV with these patients to try to avoid its use as an emergency. This therefore requires careful monitoring and assessment of patients' respiratory symptoms in order to ascertain the point at which discussions about ventilation may be appropriate and to give patients adequate time in which to think through their treatment choices.

Polkey et al. (1999) describe the ethical and clinical issues arising from the use of NIV at home for palliative care in the treatment of motor neurone disease. They recommend that respiratory failure is demonstrated by daytime hypercapnia and overnight transcutaneous oxygen saturation and carbon dioxide tension in patients for whom NIV is a consideration. They stated that patients with bulbar palsy may be less likely to tolerate NIV because of the increased risk of aspiration, but if these patients can tolerate NIV, they can derive equal benefit. However, Bourke et al. (2006) found that the advantage of using NIV applied only to those without bulbar palsy: these patients had improved survival and main-tenance or improved quality of life, while those with severe bulbar palsy had improvements in sleep-related symptoms but no survival advantage. While tracheostomy may overcome some of the difficulties of aspiration associated with bulbar palsy and allow for ease of access when suctioning, Polkey et al. (1999) suggest that tracheostomy should be avoided in these patients.

Pinto et al. (1995) compared the outcome of 10 patients with motor neurone disease treated with NIV, with 10 control patients who had refused the use of NIV. FVC in the NIV group was lower than that for the controls; however half of the NIV group were alive at 2 years com-pared with none in the control group. This highlights an important point for patients with terminal diseases – the possibility that patients may survive longer and may suffer greater degrees of disability as a result. However, research has identified that healthcare professionals may under-estimate their patient's satisfaction with their quality of life. Moss et al. (1993) identified that in 24 patients using NIV 24 hours a day via a tracheostomy due to motor neurone disease, 90% reported that they were glad they had chosen to use it, and would do so again. McDonald et al. (1996) also identified that ventilator-dependent motor neurone disease patients' scores for quality of life did not differ significantly from those not using NIV. Turkington & Elliott (2000) point out the need for healthcare professionals not to make judgements about their patients' quality of life in order to justify withholding life-supporting therapy.

End-of-life care

National initiatives regarding palliation for terminally ill breathless patients include the Liverpool Care Pathway for the Dying Patient (LCP; www.mcpcil.org.uk/liverpool_care_pathway) and the NHS End of Life Care Programme Gold Standard Framework (GSF; www. goldstandardsframework.nhs.uk). The goal of the GSF is to enable more patients to live and die where they choose so that unnecessary hospital admissions may be avoided. Much of the work revolves around improving primary care provision relating to dying at home so that appropriate local services can be commissioned. It aims to enable non-specialists in palliative care, for example GPs, community nurses (e.g. Macmillan Nurses, district nurses and community matrons), care homes and other staff, to work with specialists and hospice staff and includes any patients with any advanced illness (e.g. heart failure, COPD, frailty) in the final year or so of life as well as those in the final days.

Case study 4.5 Motor neurone disease

Adam is a 47-year-old solicitor who was diagnosed with motor neurone disease 6 months ago. He has been referred to a respiratory specialist team for assessment for home NIV in view of his deteriorating respiratory function. He is mobile but has loss of function of his upper limbs. He has been assessed by a speech and language therapist who has identified that his swallow is slow but remains intact. He can articulate with difficulty but is still able to make himself understood. His district nurse visits Adam and his wife regularly and he has regular follow-ups with a neurologist.

His arterial blood gases on room air, are:

pH	7.3
$PaCO_2$	8.76
PaO_2	7.33

Adam complains of shortness of breath on exertion. Both he and his wife understand that his disease is progressive and that the use of NIV will be palliative. He attends a 3-hour outpatient appointment to be assessed for home NIV and to learn how to use it with his wife so that both understand its function and can use it successfully. An initial arterial blood gas is taken using an earlobe sample as a baseline measure. Adam is fitted with a nasal mask and then placed on the machine. At this stage a few breaths on the machine at a time are given allowing Adam to remove it as he feels necessary, until he is comfortable enough using it to have the head gear fitted. He then tries an hour in the machine with repeat arterial blood gases at the end of that time to ensure that his arterial blood gases are not worsened by the use of the machine. A full explanation is given of how to use the machine, clean the machine and the mask and change the filters, along with contact telephone numbers and service arrangements. Discussion about end-of-life issues is also important so that relatives do not attempt to resuscitate the patient at the end of life when palliation would be more appropriate. In keeping with the palliative aims of using home NIV in this case, all alarms on the machine are turned off.

Adam uses the machine successfully at home for the next 4 months. He becomes progressively weaker and requires a suction machine at home to clear upper airway secretions. An adapted wheelchair is supplied along with a hoist at home and a battery pack to support the use of NIV outdoors. Adam dies peacefully at home in his sleep.

Contraindications

Contraindications for acute NIV

For many patients in respiratory failure, the 'gold standard' of treatment remains intubation and ventilation and the use of NIV should not replace the use of intubation and ventilation where that is the most appropriate treatment. However, where invasive ventilation is not considered appropriate but NIV would be acceptable, then a trial of NIV could be made. Contraindications to the acute use of NIV are:

- Fixed obstruction of the upper airway
- Inability to protect airway
- Life-threatening hypoxaemia
- Severe co-morbidity
- Impaired consciousness
- Confusion/agitation
- Acute asthma
- Epistaxis
- Facial trauma/burns
- Head injury/pneumoencephalos
- Allergy to masks
- Undrained pneumothorax
- Extensive bullae
- Cardiovascular instability
- Vomiting
- Bowel obstruction
- Copious respiratory secretions
- Focal consolidation on chest radiograph

The BTS guideline (2002) suggests that where NIV is the ceiling of treatment, then it could be used despite the presence of the above contraindications. However, it is not recommended in end-stage disease or where there is more than one co-morbidity present (BTS Standards of Care Committee, 2002). NIV should not be used routinely in cases of chest wall trauma; if NIV or CPAP is used in such cases, adequate monitoring must take place because of the risk of pneumothorax. It is recommended that trials of NIV for acute pneumonia and hypoxaemia resistant to high-flow oxygen should take place in the ICU or high-dependency unit (HDU) settings. NIV could be used as an alternative to tracheal intubation in cases of diffuse pneumonia who are hypoxic and hypercapnic; in this case those appropriate for intubation should receive the trial of NIV in an ICU setting.

Contraindications/precautions: home NIV

The clinical benefit to the patient must be identified by use of NIV in the inpatient setting, using arterial blood gas monitoring and polysomnography to confirm improvements in overnight arterial blood gases (Meecham-Jones et al., 1995; Simonds, 1996). In addition to the clinical assessment, the use of home NIV will also need to include a risk assessment comprising:

- Competency of the patient to manage the equipment and its use, successfully and safely.
- Patient dependence on the machine.
- How long patients could successfully spend off the machine.
- How the machine will be restored to functioning in case of breakdown within an agreed time scale.

Patients' competency should be assessed by a healthcare professional and must include an assessment of the patient's ability to turn the machine on and off and to put the mask and headgear on successfully. This can be facilitated by allowing the patient to be independent in their care towards the end of their inpatient stay. In addition, a home visit soon after discharge helps to build confidence in patients using the equipment at home and resolves any individual outstanding issues. Mikelsons et al. (2006) identified several issues that patients had concerns with when using NIV at home:

- Stigmatisation when using NIV
- Support in coming to terms with NIV
- Anxiety over using NIV

Where patients live with relatives or have carers as part of a care package, it may be possible to teach someone else about the use of the machine, with the consent of the patient. As it has been shown that patients experience feelings of stigmatisation when using this type of equipment, even in front of family members (Mikelsons et al., 2006), healthcare professionals should encourage patients to express their concerns about using the machine and find individual solutions to enable their successful use of it. It has also been shown that patients gain support from others using this type of equipment, for example in out-patient clinics, when an inpatient and at support groups. This suggests that opportunities supporting patients in exchanging their experiences should be encouraged by healthcare staff in a variety of healthcare and social settings.

A risk assessment will have identified how quickly a machine needs to be restored to functionality in case of breakdown or electrical supply problems. This may be achieved by the provision of a second machine or a machine with a battery back-up or by firms specialising in the use of NIV being contracted to supply a replacement. Electricity providers should be informed so that the supply of NIV users can be reconnected as a priority in the event of electricity failure. Written information including contact details for use in an emergency should be given to the patient.

Initiating patients on NIV successfully at home should involve patients in identifying and self-selecting care and services appropriate to their own needs (Mikelsons et al., 2006). With careful discussion between the patient and healthcare staff to ascertain and address concerns, individual requirements may be simply resolved once identified. Potential sources of support are:

- Written information including patient-held records
- One-to-one advice and education from a healthcare professional trained in home NIV
- Home visits
- A telephone helpline
- Web-based resources
- Self-help groups

An important aspect of care for these patients is advice about taking short breaks or holidays with the equipment. Patients will need practical advice about carrying and using their equipment abroad. Machines should be carried onto flights as hand luggage which may require a letter from a healthcare professional confirming its use. The use of oxygen during the flight can be arranged through the airline carrier although charges are made for this by some airlines. Most patients, but not all, using NIV will require oxygen during a long-distance flight and this requirement can be checked beforehand using a fitness to fly test, which tests a patient's response to being challenged when breathing 15% oxygen, the equivalent of breathing oxygen levels in flight at altitude. However, this will need to be done in advance with a referral for the test from a respiratory specialist physician (see Chapter 3 for more detail of travelling with oxygen). Oxygen provision at the destination can be arranged through the patient's general practitioner or specialist. Specialist advice about travel abroad with NIV and/or oxygen should be sought from healthcare professionals with specialist knowledge of this area.

Battery pack

A battery pack can be supplied in order to run a home NIV machine independently when out of the home. However, care should be taken to instruct patients and their carers in its correct use to avoid the situation where the NIV is required but the battery is flat. The manufacturer's instructions for charging and care of the battery must be followed carefully so that patients understand how many hours it takes to charge the battery and how many hours it will run for. Battery packs may also be connected to a car battery but caution should be exercised so that the car battery is not run down by the use of the NIV from it.

Application

Initiation of NIV: pre-requisites

Many members of the multi-disciplinary team have been reported to set up and maintain NIV successfully in the inpatient setting. These include medical staff, nurses, physiotherapists, clinical scientists and lung function technicians (British Thoracic Society Guidelines, 2002). A key issue in the initiation of NIV is that staff receive adequate training and keep themselves up to date in the use of the equipment and in the management of patients using it (British Thoracic Society Guidelines, 2002). This must include knowledge of machines and use of a range of masks. However, consideration should be made about the variety of equipment available, so that the range meets the needs of patients but does not result in escalating the need to re-train staff to an untenable extent.

Selection of appropriate patients for NIV should be made according to agreed criteria (BTS Standards of Care Committee, 2002). The criteria should be agreed beforehand by discussion within the multi-disciplinary team and may vary from unit to unit depending on the patient groups admitted. Within the protocols of criteria for treatment, there should also be consideration about treatment failure: this may vary from patient to patient but should be included in the management plan for the individual patient. Issues which should be addressed are:

- Patient condition deteriorates
- Failure to improve arterial blood gases
- Development of new complications
- Unable to tolerate NIV
- Failure to improve symptoms
- Deterioration in conscious level
- Patient or carer wants to stop treatment
- Resuscitation status/admission to ITU/anaesthetic opinion/ceiling of treatment

Assessment of patients

The assessment of the patient for ventilatory support in the acute setting should be thorough and careful. Patients who are being considered for this kind of support will be unwell and all patients will be in Type II respiratory failure. The referral to the anaesthetic team for intubation and ventilation should not be delayed when this is indicated. It may be necessary to consider an early referral for an anaesthetic opinion if the patient is being treated on the ward rather than in ICU or an HDU to ensure timely treatment.

A thorough assessment should be made by all members of the health-care team and all existing medical interventions should be optimised prior to initiating the use of NIV. This technique should not be used instead of other therapeutic interventions and the assessment should include all systems of the body.

Before starting NIV a pre-treatment arterial blood gas should be taken. This can be taken either via the arterial route or from the earlobe. It can be taken on room air or on added oxygen provided that a record is made of what the patient was breathing to aid future assessment. The patient should then have repeat arterial blood gases 1 hour after successful use of NIV and the two results compared.

Setting up NIV

NIV should be set up in an environment in the acute setting equipped to manage patients on NIV. More detail of suitable places in which to initiate NIV are described in Chapter 7. Application of NIV should follow the guidelines in Box 4.4. To assist staff with problem solving common issues when setting up NIV it is useful to have an action plan with the various steps required to initiate NIV with the rationale for each step (Table 4.1).

Table 4.1   Action plan for setting up NIV. With kind permission from Royal Free Hampstead NHS Trust.

Action	Rationale
Ensure ward emergency equipment available	Provide safe environment
Patient discussed with medical, nursing and physiotherapy staff	To ensure NIV is the appropriate intervention and support is available
Ensure the NIV prescription chart has been fully completed	To ensure appropriate settings are maintained
Check with medical staff that patient has a recent chest radiograph which is clear of pneumothorax/pneumonia	Pneumothorax must be discounted prior to starting NIV as positive pressure can cause lung barotrauma. If a patient already has a pneumothorax the size can be increased by NIV. NIV is unlikely to succeed if pneumonia is present
Explain procedure to patient positively and calmly. The patient will require reassurance throughout the procedure. Sit up the patient in bed	To gain consent and co-operation. This is potentially a frightening and claustrophobic experience
Set up the equipment. Ensure filter is connected to the port on the NIV machine before attaching the tubing	To prevent contamination of the machine
Carry out as much preparation as possible away from patient's bedside	To prevent distressing patient
Check size of mask which must fit firmly and not encroach on upper lip and into corners of the eye. Assess mask size using gauge on mask pack. Use nasal mask in preference to full face mask unless patient cannot keep mouth closed	To ensure seal and prevent air leaks
Apply hydrocolloid dressing to bridge of patient's nose. Check for any poor facial skin condition	This is a high-risk pressure area. Existing poor facial skin condition may also be exacerbated
Connect patient's current supplemental oxygen to second oxygen supply	Maintain oxygen supply while preparing equipment
Set to required mode and pressure settings (IPAP, EPAP) and back up BPM settings	To ensure machine is functioning correctly and that a back-up rate is provided in the spontaneous/timed mode
Turn the machine on and connect entrained oxygen to connector	To commence treatment and provide oxygen supply
Ask patient to breathe through nose and maintain tight mouth seal. Hold mask to patient's nose for a few minutes	To reassure patient and acclimatise
Attach head cap straps to mask and obtain seal. The mask should be firm but **not tight** and small leaks may be acceptable. If unable to maintain mouth seal patient may require a full face mask	To ensure no leaks
Ensure that exhalation port on connector between mask and tubing is not blocked and facing away from patient	To prevent build up of carbon dioxide
Document a set of observations	Provide baseline for assessing progress

Box 4.4   Setting up NIV.

- Decide on management plan/inform ICU
- Explain procedure to patient
- Select a mask to fit the patient and hold in place to familiarise patient
- Set up ventilator
- Start NIV allowing patient to hold mask to face for first few minutes
- Apply mask headgear, minimising leaks
- Use an oximeter to gauge response
- Remind patient not to eat or drink on the machine
- Instruct patient how to summon for help
- Make any adjustments to mask, settings
- Reassess patient and check arterial blood gases after 1 hour
- Adjust oxygen ± settings as appropriate
- If patient worse after 1 hour: stop NIV
- If no improvement, try for a further 4–6 hours and reassess, stopping if no further improvement

(Consensus Conference, 1999; BTS Standards of Care Committee, 2002)

Studies into the use of NIV for the treatment of Type II respiratory failure due to COPD have demonstrated that where there is respiratory acidosis (decreased pH) which is not corrected by ventilation the prognosis for the patient's survival is poor (Ambrosino et al., 1995). Therefore treatment with NIV should be aimed at the correction of respiratory acidosis and reducing the partial pressure of carbon dioxide in the blood.

Patients who are going to use NIV at home will have started use in hospital in most cases in order to assess the clinical benefit and also to allow the patient to gain confidence with its use. This will allow adequate education and training of the patient and relatives.

Choosing equipment (pressure and volume ventilators)

Ventilators used to deliver NIV include ICU-type ventilators with full monitoring and alarms to lighter, portable devices used specifically for delivering non-invasive ventilatory support both in the acute and domiciliary settings. Increasingly, non-invasive ventilators allow the delivery of both pre-set pressure and volume ventilation. Ideally, decisions about which mode to use would be made on the basis of the clinical requirements of each patient. However, decisions may depend on availability of equipment, experience of the team using the equipment and location of care (Evans, 2001; BTS Standards of Care Committee, 2002).

Both modes have advantages and disadvantages. Volume-targeted ventilation offers high levels of reduction in the work of breathing and constancy in terms of volume and pressure delivered but poor comfort, low trigger sensitivity and poor leak compensation compared to pressure-targeted devices. Volume-cycled machines may therefore be more appropriate for patients with changing respiratory characteristics (Evans, 2001). As peak airway pressure will not be limited in this case, these modes are more susceptible to leak which may predispose patients to gastric distension, skin necrosis and pressure sores (Evans, 2001). However, provided that respiratory characteristics are constant, then pressure support ventilation can offer reliable ventilation with high levels of patient comfort and minimal problems associated with leaks and skin necrosis (Evans, 2001).

All modes of NIV have been demonstrated to provide both physiological and clinical benefit. Appendini et al. (1994) and Vitacca et al. (2000) demonstrated improvements in minute ventilation, respiratory rate and arterial blood gases in patients with acute respiratory failure due to COPD using controlled pressure support and proportional assist modes of ventilation. Girault et al. (1999) demonstrated that both flow and pressure modes allowed respiratory muscle rest, improved breathing pattern and gas exchange when used as an extubation and weaning technique in patients with acute respiratory failure.

Ventilator features

The types of machine available for the delivery of NIV are usually either volume or pressure pre-set machines. There are a variety modes and features that the ventilators can be set on, which include:

- Assist mode
- Assist/control mode
- IPAP
- EPAP
- Inspiratory time (Ti)

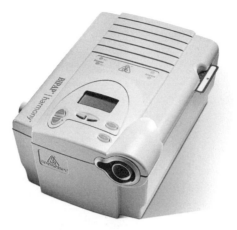

Figure 4.1 BiPAP Harmony. With kind permission from Respironics.

- Rise time
- Triggers
- Ramps

Assist mode

In the assist mode the patient can trigger breaths which are then supplied by the machine. Examples of machines with this mode are BiPAP Harmony (Figure 4.1), VPAP III and Breas Vivo 30.

Assist/control mode

The assist/control mode allows the patient to trigger their own breaths and, in addition, allows a controlled back-up respiratory rate which can be set for use in patients who hypoventilate overnight. Examples of machines with this mode are BiPAP Synchrony (Figure 4.2), VPAP III ST (Figure 4.3) and Breas Vivo 40.

Inspiratory positive airway pressure

IPAP is a feature of pressure support and pressure control ventilation. Its setting is determined by arterial blood gas results: an initial setting might be around 14–16 cmH$_2$O but this will depend on the size of the patient's chest wall and the degree of lung compliance, with larger patients requiring pressures in the region of 22–26 cmH$_2$O in order to produce change in arterial blood gases. Care should be taken when using higher levels of IPAP in the presence of emphysematous bullae,

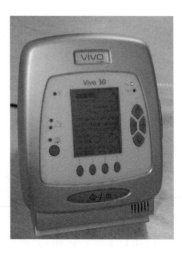

Figure 4.2   BiPAP Synchrony. With kind permission from Breas.

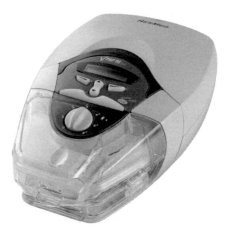

Figure 4.3   VPAP III ST. With kind permission from Resmed.

although it should be noted that emphysematous patients generally do badly on NIV, and patients with this condition should be carefully selected when considering NIV.

Expiratory positive airway pressure

The aim is to preserve a differential of at least 10 cmH_2O between IPAP and EPAP. EPAP is usually set between 4 cmH_2O and 6 cmH_2O. It helps to prevent re-breathing of carbon dioxide by prolonging gaseous exchange, enables the recruitment of alveoli and increases functional residual capacity. It offsets the inspiratory threshold load which occurs in the presence of severe COPD and is caused by the patient's intrinsic positive end expiratory pressure (PEEPi). It is thought that it reduces the inspiratory work required to trigger inspiration in patients with PEEPi and reduces the pressure change required which has to be overcome in order for pressure and flow change to occur.

Inspiratory time

Each type of machine has its own pressure characteristics which determine the speed of delivery of the breath from the machine. In some machines this can be altered by using an inspiratory time feature which allows the speed of delivery of the breath to be varied. This is usually set at 1–1.5 seconds. Adequate ventilation may be made more effective by fine tuning this setting, as if the machine is set to deliver a quick rise in pressure in a patient who has high airway pressures and non-compliant lungs, efficient ventilation may not be achieved. In this case a setting delivering a slower inspiratory time (e.g. 2 seconds) may be more efficient in ventilating the patient.

Rise time

Some machines allow patients to set a rise time (i.e. the time it takes to cycle between EPAP and IPAP) to maximise their comfort.

Triggers

Triggers should ensure that respiratory muscles do not become fatigued as they should be sensitive enough to reduce the work of breathing. A sensitive trigger enables a quick response time in delivery of the breath to the patient. If the trigger is not sensitive enough the patient has to struggle for a triggered breath thereby increasing the work of breathing. Some non-invasive ventilators have a pre-set trigger while others allow the trigger to be altered (e.g. NIPPY ST+, Figure 4.4).

Ramps

Some machines enable the setting of a ramp which allows a progressive build up to the pre-set inspiratory pressure, determined by the operator. This can be used where patients find the pre-set inspiratory pressure uncomfortable in the first few breaths and can help in maximising acceptance of the machine.

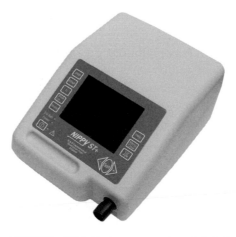

Figure 4.4 NIPPY ST+. With kind permission from B & D Electromedical.

Choosing equipment (interfaces)

The choice of mask for delivering NIV is important in order to fully optimise ventilation – mask leak is high on the list of complications described by Meduri et al. (1996) and Hill (2002). In addition failure rates of between 10% and 40% with NIV have been identified (Brochard et al., 1995; Kramer et al., 1995; Meduri, et al., 1996; Celikel et al., 1998). Studies have described the successful use of a variety of mask types:

- Face mask
- Nasal mask
- Full face mask
- Mini-mask
- Nasal pillows
- Mouthpiece

The use of a face mask (Figure 4.5) has the advantage that it can enable delivery of higher ventilatory pressures, higher minute ventilation and as a result may produce lower $PaCO_2$ compared to those achieved when using a nasal mask (Navalesi et al., 2000). It requires less patient co-operation, which may be useful if patients cannot form an adequate seal with their mouth. However, it may increase claustrophobia and gastric distension.

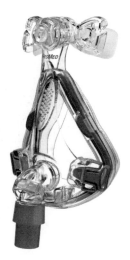

Figure 4.5   Ultra Mirage Quattro face mask. With kind permission from Resmed.

The disadvantages when using a face mask are that it may be less comfortable, it impedes communication more than a nasal mask, and limits oral intake and sputum clearance.

Nasal masks

Nasal masks (Figure 4.6) are better tolerated than face masks (Navalesi et al., 2000) with decreased claustrophobia. They allow for communication,

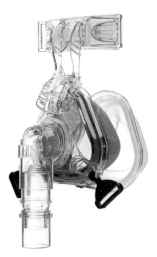

Figure 4.6   Comfort gel nasal mask. With kind permission from Respironics.

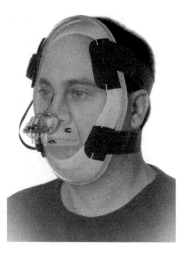

Figure 4.7   Total face mask. With kind permission from Respironics.

oral intake and sputum clearance but do require a patent nasal airway
and for patients to be able to keep their mouth closed.

Evans (2001) recommended that both full face and nasal masks
are useful with no evidence to support the use of a particular device.
The BTS guideline (2002) suggests the use of a full face mask in an acute
setting for the first 24 hours with the option to change to a nasal mask as
the patient improves.

Full face mask

Full face masks (Figure 4.7) can be used for patients who are claustrophobic when using a nasal or face mask as they cover the entire face
forming a seal around the hair line and jaw. Criner et al. (1994) found
patients were able to achieve acceptable results using the device.

Mini-mask

Mini-masks (Figure 4.8) provide another alternative for those suffering
from claustrophobia and cover the tip of the nose only. Most come with
a built-in exhale valve and therefore should only be used with pressure
support machines. Examples of mini-masks are Simplicity (Respironics)
and Phantom (Sleepnet).

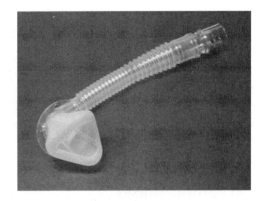

Figure 4.8   Simplicity mini mask. With kind permission from Respironics.

Nasal pillows

Traditionally nasal pillows (Figure 4.9) were used in the delivery of continuous positive airway pressure (CPAP) for the treatment of obstructive sleep apnoea but more recently have become popular for the delivery of NIV. They have the same application as mini-masks but apply ventilation through two pillows which rest next to the nares forming a seal.

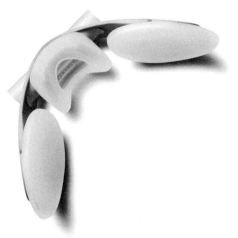

Figure 4.9   Comfort curve head nasal pillows. With kind permission from Respironics.

Mouthpieces

Bach (1997) describes the successful use of mouthpieces for the delivery of NIV in patients with neuromuscular disease such as muscular dystrophy. However, a patient using this type of device must be able to form a seal with their mouth in order to receive adequate ventilation. In addition care should be taken with dental care as front teeth may become loosened with prolonged use.

Prevention of complications

The incidence of complications with the use of NIV can be high, with a failure rate of between 10% and 40% (Brochard et al., 1995; Kramer et al., 1995; Meduri et al., 1996; Celikel et al., 1998). The issues which have been identified by Soo Hoo et al. (1994) as contributors to failure are:

- Edentulate
- Pneumonia
- Sputum retention
- Poor mouth seal
- Greater mouth leaks

Mask leaks can be a major problem and may be significant during sleep (Teschler et al., 1999; Navalesi et al., 2000). Meduri et al. (1996) and Hill (2002) studied the incidence of complications, which include:

- Mask leak
- Facial skin necrosis
- Conjunctivitis
- Gastric distention
- Sputum retention
- Pneumonia

Troubleshooting

Mask leak

Mask leaks should be resolved quickly to ensure re-establishment of effective ventilation. This may require refitting or changing to an alternative mask depending on the problem and a range of masks should be available to allow for this.

Pressure sores

Pressure sores should be dealt with as a matter of urgency as skin necrosis could impact on the patient's ability to accept NIV. In addition, where NIV is the ceiling of treatment, it may not be appropriate to offer alternative supplementary interventions. A number of hydrocolloid dressings are available which can be cut to fit the glabellar (bridge) region of the nose which is the area most likely to breakdown (Callaghan & Trapp, 1998). Other solutions include the use of a Silastic prosthesis (Meecham-Jones et al., 1994) which can be fitted to sit between the face and the mask. Masks can also be lined with self-adhesive towelling. More recently, gel masks have been developed, which have the advantage of moulding to the contours of the face when warmed by the patient's skin.

Abdominal distension

Abdominal distension can be a source of discomfort for patients and may be caused by swallowing of air delivered by the machine which may be resolved by explaining that patients should allow the machine to do the work rather than swallowing the breaths delivered. Charcoal biscuits available from health food shops and carbonated drinks are also helpful in reducing distension.

Sputum retention

The presence of sputum will prevent adequate ventilation and must be treated effectively using interventions such as physiotherapy, humidification, nebulisers, oral fluids and antibiotics.

Rhinitis

Some patients experience rhinitis on using NIV which can be treated with nasal decongestants or if these do not help then humidification may be added into the NIV circuit.

Claustrophobia

Claustrophobia can be an issue for some and alternative masks such as mini-masks, or full face masks (Respironics) (Criner et al., 1994) may be the alternatives of choice.

Transient hypoxaemia

Transient hypoxaemia should be monitored carefully so that patients receive adequate support at all times. Monitoring can be achieved simply by using an oximeter: however, all team members should be aware of the appropriate steps to take in response to a patient's falling oxygen saturation.

Nutrition

Adequate nutrition for patients receiving NIV should be addressed using a fine bore nasogastric tube if patients require long periods of NIV. Once a patient is more stable then regular periods off NIV should be encouraged and oral intake resumed.

References

Ambrosino, N., Foglio, K., Rubini, F., Clini, E., Nava, S. & Vitacca, M. (1995) Non-invasive mechanical ventilation in acute respiratory failure due to chronic obstructive pulmonary disease: correlates for success. *Thorax*, **50** (7), 755–757.

Antonelli, M., Conti, G., Rocco, M., Bufi, M., De Blasi, R.A., Vivino, G., Gasparetto, A. & Meduri, G.U. (1998) A comparison of non-invasive positive pressure ventilation and conventional mechanical ventilation in patients with acute respiratory failure. *New England Journal of Medicine*, **339** (7), 429–435.

Appendini, L., Patessio, A., Zanaboni, S., Carone, M., Gukov, B., Donner, C.F., Rossi, A. (1994) Physiologic effects of positive end-expiratory pressure and mask pressure support during exacerbations of chronic obstructive pulmonary disease. *American Journal of Respiratory and Critical Care Medicine*, **149**, 1069–1076.

Bach, J.R. (1997) The prevention of ventilatory failure due to inadequate pump function. *Respiratory Care*, **42** (4), 403–413.

Barbé, F., Togores, B., Rubí, M., Pons, S., Maimó, A. & Agustí, A.G. (1996) Noninvasive ventilatory support does not facilitate recovery from acute respiratory failure in chronic obstructive pulmonary disease. *European Respiratory Journal*, **9**, 1240–1245.

Bott, J., Baudouin, S.V. & Moxham, J. (1991) Nasal intermittent positive pressure ventilation in the treatment of respiratory failure in obstructive sleep apnoea. *Thorax*, **46**, 457–458.

Bott, J., Carroll, M.P., Conway, J.H., et al. (1993) Randomised controlled trial of nasal ventilation in acute ventilatory failure due to chronic obstructive airways disease. *Lancet*, **341**, 1555–1557.

Bourke, S.C., Tomlinson, M., Williams, T.L., Bullock, R.E., Shaw, P.J. & Gibson, G.J. (2006) Effects of non-invasive ventilation on survival and quality of life in patients with amyotrophic lateral sclerosis: a randomised controlled trial. *Lancet Neurology*, **5** (4), 291–292.

British Thoracic Society Standards of Care Committee (2002) BTS Guideline. Non-invasive ventilation in acute respiratory failure. *Thorax*, **57**, 192–211.

Brochard, L., Mancebo, J., Wysocki, M. et al. (1995) Noninvasive ventilation for acute exacerbations of chronic obstructive pulmonary disease. *New England Journal of Medicine*, **333**, 817–822.

Callaghan, S. & Trapp, M. (1998) Evaluating two dressings for the prevention of nasal bridge pressure sores. *Professional Nurse*, **13**, 361–364.

Casanova, C., Celli, B.R., Tost, L., Soriano, E., Abreu, J., Velasco, V. & Santolaria, F. (2000) Long-term controlled trial of nocturnal nasal positive pressure ventilation in patients with severe COPD. *Chest*, **118** (6), 1582–1590.

Celikel, T., Sungur, M., Ceyhan, B. et al. (1998) Comparison of non-invasive positive pressure ventilation with standard medical therapy in hypercapnic acute respiratory failure. *Chest*, **114**, 1636–1642.

Chu, C.M., Chan, V.L., Lin, A.W., Wong, I.W., Leung, W.S. & Lai, C.K. (2004) Readmission rates and life threatening events in COPD survivors treated with non-invasive ventilation for acute hypercapnic respiratory failure. *Thorax*, **59** (12), 1020–1025.

Clini, E., Sturani, C., Rossi, A., Viaggi, S., Corrado, A., Donner, C.F. & Ambrosino, N. (2002) The Italian multicentre study on non-invasive ventilation in chronic obstructive pulmonary disease patients. *European Respiratory Journal*, **20**, 529–538.

Consensus Conference (1999) Clinical indications for non-invasive positive pressure ventilation in chronic respiratory failure due to restrictive lung disease. *Chest*, **116**, 521–534.

Criner, G.J., Travaline, J.M., Brennan, K.J. & Kreimer, D.T. (1994) Efficacy of a new full face mask for non-invasive positive pressure ventilation. *Chest*, **106**, 1109–1115.

Ellis, E.R., Grunstein, R.R., Chan, C.S., Bye, P.T.P. & Sullivan, C.E. (1988) Treatment of nocturnal respiratory failure in kyphoscoliosis. *Chest*, **94**, 811–815.

Evans, T.W. (2001) International Consensus Conference in Intensive Care Medicine: Non-invasive positive pressure ventilation in acute respiratory failure. *Intensive Care Medicine*, **27**, 166–178.

Girault, C., Daudenthun, I., Chevron, V., Tamion, F., Leroy, J. & Bonmarchand, G. (1999) Non-invasive ventilation as systematic extubation and weaning technique in acute on chronic respiratory failure. *American Journal of Respiratory and Critical Care*, **160**, 86–92.

Gozal, D. (1997) Nocturnal ventilatory support in patients with cystic fibrosis: comparison with supplemental oxygen. *European Respiratory Journal*, **10** (9), 1999–2003.

Hill, A.T., Edenborough, F.P., Cayton, R.M. & Stableforth, D.E. (1998) Long term nasal intermittent positive pressure ventilation in patients with Cystic Fibrosis and hypercapnic respiratory failure (1991–1996). *Respiratory Medicine*, **92** (3), 523–526.

Hill, N.S. (2002) Saving face: better interfaces for non-invasive ventilation. *Intensive Care Medicine*, **28**, 227–229.

Hodson, M.E., Madden, B.P., Steven, M.H., Tsang, V.T. & Yacoub, M.H. (1991) Non-invasive mechanical ventilation for cystic fibrosis patients – a potential bridge to transplantation. *European Respiratory Journal*, **4**, 524–527.

Kerby, G.R., Mayer, L.S. & Pingleton, S.K. (1987) Nocturnal positive pressure ventilation via a nasal mask. *American Journal of Respiratory Disease*, **135**, 738–740.

Kramer, N., Meyer, T.J., Mehang, J., Cece, R.D. & Hill, N.S. (1995) Randomized, prospective trial of noninvasive positive pressure ventilation in acute respiratory failure. *American Journal of Respiratory and Critical Care Medicine*, **151**, 1799–1806.

Leger, P., Bedicam, J.M., Cornette, A., Reybet-Degat, O. & Langevin, B. (1994) Nasal intermittent positive pressure ventilation. *Chest*, **105**, 100–105.

Lloyd-Owen, S.J., Donaldson, G.C., Ambrosino, N. et al. (2005) Patterns of home mechanical ventilation use in Europe: results from the Eurovent survey. *European Respiratory Journal*, **25**, 1025–1031.

Madden, B.P., Kariyawasam, H., Siddiqi, A.J., Machin, A., Pryor, J.A. & Hodson, M.E. (2002). Noninvasive ventilation in cystic fibrosis patients with acute or chronic respiratory failure. *European Respiratory Journal*, **19** (2), 310–313.

Masip, J., Betbese, A.J. & Paez, J. (2000) Non-invasive pressure support ventilation versus conventional oxygen therapy in acute cardiogenic pulmonary oedema: a randomised trial. *Lancet*, **356**, 2126–2132.

McDonald, E.R., Hillel, A. & Wiedenfeld, S.A. (1996) Evaluation of the psychological status of ventilatory-supported patients with ALS/MND. *Palliative Medicine*, **10** (1), 35–41.

Meduri, G.U., Turner, R.E., Abou-Shala, N., Wunderink, R. & Tolley, E. (1996) Non-invasive positive-pressure ventilation via face mask: first-line intervention in patients with acute hypercapnic and hypoxemic respiratory failure. *Chest*, **109**, 179–193.

Meecham-Jones, D.J., Braid, G. & Wedzicha, J.A. (1994) Nasal masks for domiciliary positive pressure ventilation: patient usage and complications. *Thorax*, **49**, 811–812.

Meecham-Jones, D.J., Paul, E.A., Jones, P.W. & Wedzicha, J.A. (1995) Nasal pressure support ventilation plus oxygen compared with oxygen therapy alone in hypercapnic COPD. *American Journal of Respiratory and Critical Care Medicine*, **152**, 538–544.

Mikelsons, C., Muncey, T. & Wedzicha, J.A. (2006) Experience of chronic obstructive pulmonary disease patients using home non-invasive ventilation. *Thorax*, **61** (Suppl 2), ii57–ii133 (P182).

Moss, A., Casey, P., Stocking, C. et al. (1993) Home ventilation for amyotrophic lateral sclerosis patients. *Neurology*, **43**, 438–443.

National Institute for Clinical Excellence (2004) Chronic Obstructive Pulmonary Disease. National clinical guideline on management of chronic pulmonary disease in adults in primary and secondary care. *Thorax*, **59** (Suppl 1), 1–232.

Nava, S., Ambrosino, N., Clini, E. et al. (1998) Noninvasive mechanical ventilation in the weaning of patients with respiratory failure due to chronic obstructive pulmonary disease. A randomised controlled trial. *Annals of Internal Medicine*, **128**, 721–728.

Navalesi, P., Fanfulla, F., Frigerio, P., Gregoretti, C. & Nava, S. (2000) Physiologic evaluation of noninvasive mechanical ventilation delivered with three types of masks in patients with chronic hypercapnic respiratory failure. *Critical Care Medicine*, **28** (6), 1785–1790.

Pang, D., Keenan, S.P., Cook, D.J. & Sibbald, W.J. (1998) The effect of positive pressure airway support in mortality and the need for intubation in cardiogenic pulmonary oedema: a systematic review. *Chest*, **114**, 1185–1192.

Pinto, A.C., Evangelista, T., Carvalho, M., Alves, M.A. & Sales Luís, M.L. (1995) Respiratory assistance with a non-invasive ventilator (BiPAP) in MND/ALS patients: survival rates in a controlled trial. *Journal of Neurological Science*, **129**, 19–26.

Piper, A.J., Parker, S., Torzillo, P.J., Sullivan, C.E. & Bye, P.T. (1992) Nocturnal nasal IPPV stabilizes patients with cystic fibrosis and hypercapnic respiratory failure. *Chest*, **102** (3), 846–850.

Plant, P.K., Owen, J.L. & Elliott, M.W. (2000) Early use of non-invasive ventilation for acute exacerbations of chronic obstructive pulmonary disease on general respiratory wards: a multicentre randomised controlled trial. *Lancet*, **355**, 1931–1935.

Polkey, M.I., Lyall, R.A., Davidson, C.A. et al. (1999) Ethical and clinical issues in the use of home non-invasive mechanical ventilation for the palliation of breathlessness in motor neurone disease. *Thorax*, **54** (4), 367–371.

Ram, F.S.F., Lightowler, J.V. & Wedzicha, J.A. (2003) Non-invasive ventilation for treatment of respiratory failure due to exacerbations of chronic pulmonary disease. In: *The Cochrane Library*, Issue 3. Oxford: Update Software.

Respiratory Alliance (2003) *Bridging the Gap*. Direct Publishing Solutions, Cookham.

Restrick, L.J., Scott, A.D., Ward, A.D., Feneck, R.O., Cornwell, W.E. & Wedzicha, J.A. (1993) Nasal intermittent positive-pressure ventilation in weaning intubated patients with chronic respiratory disease from assisted intermittent positive-pressure ventilation. *Respiratory Medicine*, **87**, 199–204.

Seneff, M.G., Wagner, D.P., Wagner, R.P., Zimmerman, J.E. & Knaus, W.A. (1995) Hospital and 1-year survival of patients admitted to intensive care units with acute exacerbation of chronic obstructive pulmonary disease. *Journal of the American Medical Association*, **274**, 1852–1857.

Sharon, A., Shpirer, I., Kaluski, E. et al. (2000) High dose intravenous isosorbide-dinitrate is safer and better than BiPAP ventilation combined with conventional treatment for severe pulmonary oedema. *Journal of the American College of Cardiology*, **36**, 832–837.

Simonds, A.K. (1996) *Non-invasive Respiratory Support*. 1st edn. Chapman & Hall, London.

Simonds, A.K. & Elliott, M.W. (1995) Outcome of domiciliary nasal intermittent positive pressure ventilation in restrictive and obstructive disorders. *Thorax*, **50**, 604–609.

Simonds, A.K., Muntoni, F., Heather, S. & Fielding, S. (1998) Impact of nasal ventilation on survival in hypercapnic Duchenne muscular dystrophy. *Thorax*, **53** (11), 949–952.

Sivasothy, P., Smith, I.E. & Shneerson, J.M. (1998) Mask intermittent positive pressure ventilation in chronic hypercapnic respiratory failure due to chronic obstructive pulmonary disease. *European Respiratory Journal*, **11**, 34–40.

Soo Hoo, G.W., Santiago, S. & Williams, A.J. (1994) Nasal mechanical ventilation for hypercapnic respiratory failure in chronic obstructive pulmonary disease: determinants of success and failure. *Critical Care Medicine*, **22**, 1253–1261.

Sullivan, C.E., Berthon-Jones, M., Issa, F.G. & Eves, L. (1981) Reversal of obstructive sleep apnoea by continuous positive airway pressure applied through the nose. *Lancet*, **i**, 862–865.

Teschler, H., Stampa, J., Ragette, R., Konietzko, N. & Berthon-Jones, M. (1999) Effect of mouth leak on effctiveness of nasal bilevel ventilatory assistance and sleep architecture. *European Respiratory Journal*, **14**, 1251–1257.

Tuggey, J.M., Plant, P.K. & Elliott, M.W. (2003) Domiciliary non-invasive ventilation for recurrent acidotic exacerbations of COPD: an economic analysis. *Thorax*, **58**, 867–871.

Turkington, P.M. & Elliott, M.W. (2000) Rationale for the use of non-invasive ventilation in chronic ventilatory failure. *Thorax*, **55** (5), 417–423.

Udwadia, Z.F., Santis, G.F., Steven, M.H. & Simonds, A.K. (1992) Nasal ventilation to facilitate weaning in patients with chronic respiratory insufficiency. *Thorax*, **47** (9), 715–718.

Vitacca, M., Clini, E., Pagani, M., Bianchi, L., Rossi, A. & Ambrosino, N. (2000) Physiologic effects of early administered mask proportional assist ventilation in patients with chronic obstructive pulmonary disease and acute respiratory failure. *Critical Care Medicine*, **28** (6), 1791–1797.

Chapter 5

CONTINUOUS POSITIVE AIRWAY PRESSURE (CPAP)

Continuous positive airway pressure (CPAP) is the use of positive airway pressure applied throughout the respiratory cycle, delivered to the spontaneously breathing patient for therapeutic reasons. CPAP can take two forms, each of which has different indications and applications in the clinical setting. CPAP generated by a flow generator in the acute setting is used as a form of respiratory support in the treatment of Type I respiratory failure. CPAP generated by an electrically powered motor is used to treat obstructive sleep apnoea in the domiciliary setting. It is important to understand the distinct use of each type of therapy as they are not interchangeable and should be used in different clinical circumstances.

CPAP for the treatment of Type I respiratory failure

Principles of treatment

CPAP for the treatment of Type I respiratory failure delivers high levels of oxygen and is created by a flow generator attached to an oxygen supply. The oxygen is delivered to the patients by means of a face mask, nasal mask, hood, mouth piece, or tracheostomy. The expiratory pressures are set above atmospheric pressure and therefore both inspiratory and expiratory pressures are increased (American Association of Respiratory Care (AARC), 1993; Figure 5.1).

As patients are spontaneously breathing during CPAP, both respiratory rate and tidal volume are determined by the patient; hence CPAP should be viewed as a respiratory rather than a ventilatory support as ventilatory parameters, such as tidal or minute volume, remain unchanged by the use of CPAP. This is an important point for consideration when using CPAP therapeutically because it may not result in a change in $PaCO_2$. The therapeutic use of CPAP relies on the delivery of

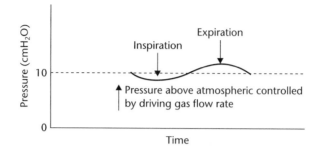

Figure 5.1   Profile of continuous positive airway pressure (CPAP) pressures.

a high flow of oxygen (fraction of inspired oxygen (FiO$_2$) of 35–90%) creating positive airway pressures which splint open alveoli during the expiratory phase of respiration allowing longer time for gaseous exchange. This results in the physiological effects outlined below (Stock et al., 1985; Lindner et al., 1987; Bersten et al., 1991; AARC, 1993; Lin et al., 1995; Mehta et al., 1997; British Thoracic Society (BTS) Standards of Care Committee, 2002).

The physiological effects of high-flow CPAP are:

- Increased oxygenation
- Increased functional residual capacity
- Improved ventilation–perfusion matching
- Improved collateral ventilation
- Improved sputum clearance
- Decreased work of breathing
- Reduction in pre-load and after load

Indications

The main indication for the use of CPAP is hypoxaemia as a result of Type I respiratory failure. This can be the result of a cardiogenic or a pulmonary cause and CPAP can be a useful adjunct to treatment in either case. However, it is important to understand the underlying clinical cause of the hypoxaemia so that other appropriate medical interventions can be started. Clinical indications for the use of CPAP are:

- Type I respiratory failure
- Pneumonia
- Post-operative atelectasis
- Acute cardiogenic pulmonary oedema

- Chest wall trauma
- Sputum retention

The use of CPAP in the treatment of cardiogenic pulmonary oedema has been shown to reduce the rate of endotracheal intubation, improve oxygenation and hypercapnia, and a trend to reduced mortality (Bersten et al., 1991; Lin et al., 1995; Mehta et al., 1997; Winck et al., 2006). Comparisons of the use of non-invasive ventilation (NIV) with CPAP in the treatment of acute cardiogenic pulmonary oedema have produced conflicting results (Mehta et al., 1997; Park et al., 2001; Martin-Bermudez et al., 2002; Bellone et al., 2004; Crane et al., 2004; Park et al., 2004; Bellone et al., 2005). Both treatments decreased the need to intubate and mortality compared with standard medical therapy, but the difference between the two has been shown to be non-significant. Winck et al. (2006) there-fore concluded that CPAP should be considered in preference to NIV as it is cheaper and easier to implement in the clinical setting. However, NIV may be used for cardiogenic pulmonary oedema if there is co-existent Type II respiratory failure or where CPAP has proved to be ineffective (BTS Standards of Care Committee, 2002). A randomised controlled trial of the use of CPAP for the treatment of chest wall trauma compared CPAP with invasive positive pressure ventilation (IPPV) (Bolliger & Van Eeden, 1990). All of the patients included in the study had a $PaO_2 > 8$ kPa with an FiO_2 of 40%. The study showed a reduction in the mean duration of treatment, reduced mean number of days spent in the intensive care unit (ICU), decreased period of hospitalisation and fewer complications when CPAP was compared with mechanical ventilation. It demonstrated that the use of CPAP for patients with chest trauma can shorten and simplify treatment.

Equipment

Various systems are available for the delivery of CPAP. These include: high-flow closed systems, which may delivery continuous or demand flow, or open systems, such as the Boussignac system, which are suit-able for short-term use only (i.e. <24 hours). The selection of appropriate high-flow system must consider a number of important factors:

- Complexity of use
- Effectiveness
- Transportability
- Number of components
- Expense

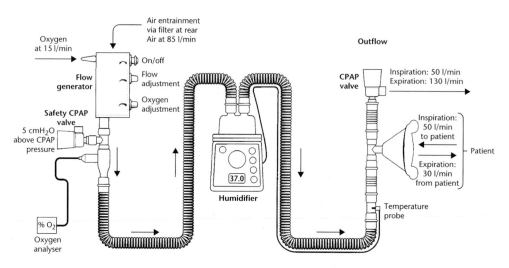

Figure 5.2   Humidified CPAP circuit. With kind permission from Respironics.

Decisions about which system to use must be based on the type of patient who may need the intervention, where treatment will take place, the resources available to provide the service and the training needs of staff providing the service.

The circuit used for CPAP must be set up according to the manufacturer's guidelines (Figure 5.2). Inclusion of a second safety CPAP valve (positive end-expiratory pressure valve (PEEP)) at the flow generator end of the circuit ensures that should the treatment CPAP valve (at the patient end of the circuit) malfunction, then the circuit will continue to remain functional.

High-flow closed systems

CPAP systems which delivery high flows do so via a flow generator (e.g. Whisperflow, Respironics) which requires connection to a wall supply of oxygen in order to deliver oxygen flows at 80–100 l/min. Gas flows through the system continuously throughout the respiratory cycle. As a result these systems can be noisy, but they can be made quieter by attaching a filter to the air inlet port.

High-flow demand systems

CPAP systems that deliver on demand rather than continuous flow systems can be used. These systems allow gas to flow only on initiation by the patient. These systems may use less gas and be less noisy than the

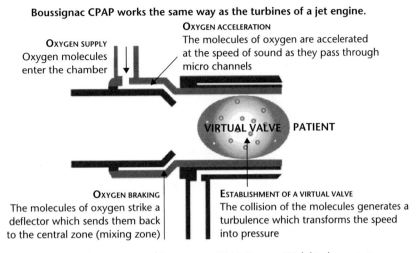

Boussignac CPAP works the same way as the turbines of a jet engine.

OXYGEN SUPPLY
Oxygen molecules
enter the chamber

OXYGEN ACCELERATION
The molecules of oxygen are accelerated
at the speed of sound as they pass through
micro channels

VIRTUAL VALVE PATIENT

OXYGEN BRAKING
The molecules of oxygen strike a
deflector which sends them back
to the central zone (mixing zone)

ESTABLISHMENT OF A VIRTUAL VALVE
The collision of the molecules generates a
turbulence which transforms the speed
into pressure

Figure 5.3 Diagram of Boussignac CPAP System. With kind permission
from Vitaid.

continuous flow systems, but they may increase the patient's work of
breathing. Both systems require several component parts, knowledge
of assembly and settings, high flows of piped oxygen or air, and have
limited transportability.

Open CPAP systems

A recent alternative to the high-flow systems is the open system,
e.g. Boussignac (Figure 5.3). This system is suitable for short-term use
only (i.e. <24 hours). It is inexpensive, eliminates capital investment in
equipment and repair, is easily transportable and allows rapid set up.
However, there is limited evidence describing its use and the system
delivers uncontrolled levels of oxygen.

Initiation of CPAP and manipulation of settings

Before starting CPAP, adequate assessment of the patient must be
carried out and the clinical indications for CPAP firmly established.
Only patients with Type I respiratory failure should be commenced on
CPAP. Identification of patients' needs for this supportive intervention should be pro-active rather than reactive as this may well prevent
further escalation to more invasive treatment options such as ventilation via endotracheal tube. This is an important consideration for the
outcome of patient care as intubation carries with it high levels of

ventilator-associated pneumonia and mortality. Assessment of the patient must include all systems of the body including the respiratory system, with particular reference to those factors which are indicators for the use of CPAP listed below, as well as any risk factors which may contribute to respiratory failure, such as:

- Hypoxaemia requiring $FiO_2 > 60\%$
- Respiratory rate >25
- Use of accessory muscles, e.g. sternocleidomastoid, trapezius
- Signs of fatigue, e.g. sweating
- Drowsiness or confusion as result of hypoxaemia

Risk factors which may contribute to Type I respiratory failure are:

- Major surgery
- Obesity
- Advancing age
- Previous history of heavy smoking
- Pre-existing respiratory disease, e.g. COPD

Initial start pressures for the PEEP treatment valve should be decided taking into account the clinical picture of the patient and according to patient tolerance. Higher PEEP pressures may be required in patients who have higher levels of hypoxaemia or who have a large chest wall. In patients who are unable to tolerate CPAP delivered by face mask, alternatives such as the nasal mask, helmet or mouthpiece can be used.

The effects of CPAP must be monitored at regular intervals; in all cases, patients requiring CPAP will be more highly dependent than those requiring 'routine' care. Re-assessment should include the following factors (AARC Guidelines, 1993):

- Patient's subjective response (pain, discomfort, dyspnoea, response to therapy, reduction in requirement for CPAP)
- Pulse rate, blood pressure, respiratory rate
- Improvements in oxygenation – SpO_2 (pulse oximeter oxygen saturation) and arterial blood gases
- Skin colour, cyanosis
- Breathing pattern, work of breathing, tidal volume, breath sounds
- Sputum production (quantity, colour, consistency, odour)
- Intracranial pressure (ICP) – in whom this is of critical importance
- Gastric distension – consider nasogastric tube to decompress stomach
- Skin patency – consider use of a hydrocolloid dressing

- Mask leak
- Oral hygiene
- Hydration

The CPAP system should be checked to confirm that the correct levels of oxygen and PEEP are delivered and that there are minimal leaks in the circuit.

Contraindications

Contraindications for the use of CPAP include (AARC, 1993):

- Facial trauma
- Basal skull fracture
- Epistaxis
- Uncontrolled emesis
- Unconscious level with inability to protect airway
- Undrained pneumothorax
- Haemodynamic stability
- Patient intolerance
- Asthma
- Type II respiratory failure as a result of COPD
- Poor patient–mask interface with large leak
- Bullae
- Lung abscess
- Severe haemoptysis
- Bronchial tumour in proximal airway
- Post-operative air leak
- Hypotension

CPAP and physiotherapy

The use of high-flow CPAP as an adjunct to physiotherapy has been described in the literature (Pryor & Prasad, 2002). In this instance, CPAP is used as a means of re-expanding atelectatic areas of lung or in aiding collateral ventilation and therefore sputum clearance. CPAP is incorporated into the active cycle of breathing techniques with the patient being encouraged to perform tidal breaths followed by lower thoracic expansion exercises while on the CPAP. Alternatively, CPAP can be used intermittently again as part of physiotherapy. In this case CPAP might be given for a period of 10–15 minutes every hour again to re-expand atelectatic areas of lung or to aid sputum clearance. However, it is important to note that the effect of CPAP is lost as soon as the CPAP mask is removed.

Trouble shooting

Setting pressures

PEEP pressures may need to be reviewed when hypoxaemia is not corrected with initial settings. PEEP pressures can be increased to a maximum of 20 cmH$_2$O but most patients will be started on 5–10 cmH$_2$O. However, before starting treatment at these high pressures, haemodynamic stability needs careful assessment as increased intrathoracic pressures caused by high levels of PEEP could result in hypotension.

Titrating FiO$_2$

The FiO$_2$ should be titrated using the results of arterial blood gases to guide the level of supplemental oxygen. The levels of oxygen delivered are determined by the use of the oxygen analyser in the CPAP circuit. Patients should receive adequate oxygenation but should not be hyper-oxygenated as this too can be harmful in the long term (Downs, 2003).

Humidification

In patients with tenacious secretions it may be necessary to deliver humidified humidification with the CPAP. Effective humidification can be given by using a T piece to entrain humidified air into the CPAP circuit. Systems capable of providing adequate humidification in the presence of high flows of gas must be used.

Weaning

Weaning from CPAP should be performed in a timely manner: there is little benefit for patients in being over-treated. The following criteria can be used to determine when weaning is appropriate:

- Absence of respiratory distress.
- SpO$_2$ > 94% for <70 years of age and >92% for >70 years of age.
- Intermittent usage of CPAP only.

- Reduced need for high inspired oxygen concentration.
- CPAP PEEP levels reduced.

There are a number of ways of weaning from CPAP:

- Reduction of FiO_2.
- Reduction of PEEP pressure.
- Intermittent use of CPAP with greater lengths of time between usage.

A guideline for decreasing the FiO_2 would be reduction in steps of 0.1 (10%) until an FiO_2 of 0.4 (40%) is reached. PEEP pressures could be reduced in increments of 2.5 cmH_2O until a PEEP pressure of 5.0 cmH_2O is reached. Intermittent use of CPAP may consist of applying CPAP for 2 hours at a time, with a break of 1 hour before the next application. In all cases, adequate monitoring should be done to determine the effect of the decrease in support. The time frame for weaning from CPAP will be dependent on the indications for its use and on the individual patient's parameters.

On-going care

In all instances where CPAP has been used, once patients have been weaned from it they must be followed up to ensure continuation of recovery. Patients may have been cared for in a number of settings which could include the intensive care unit, high dependency unit or in the ward setting. Wherever CPAP therapy is given, adequate monitoring and continuing care must be provided. Continuing care should include regular assessment of all systems as described previously. Risk factors even in the absence of the need for CPAP should also be considered. This may be done by any healthcare professional who has knowledge, skills and training in caring for patients using CPAP.

Service delivery

Initiating CPAP protocol

Safe delivery of CPAP therapy should follow a pre-determined protocol which takes into account local conditions and practices. This will allow a description of pre-conditions that should be met prior to instituting

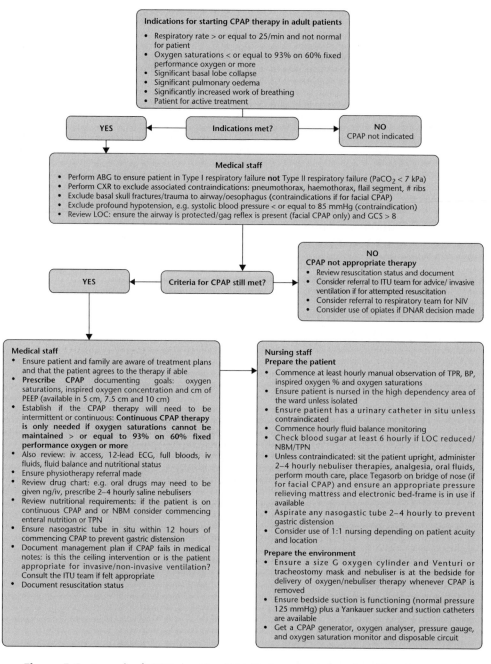

Indications for starting CPAP therapy in adult patients

- Respiratory rate > or equal to 25/min and not normal for patient
- Oxygen saturations < or equal to 93% on 60% fixed performance oxygen or more
- Significant basal lobe collapse
- Significant pulmonary oedema
- Significantly increased work of breathing
- Patient for active treatment

YES ← **Indications met?** → **NO** CPAP not indicated

Medical staff
- Perform ABG to ensure patient in Type I respiratory failure **not** Type II respiratory failure (PaCO$_2$ < 7 kPa)
- Perform CXR to exclude associated contraindications: pneumothorax, haemothorax, flail segment, # ribs
- Exclude basal skull fractures/trauma to airway/oesophagus (contraindications if for facial CPAP)
- Exclude profound hypotension, e.g. systolic blood pressure < or equal to 85 mmHg (contraindication)
- Review LOC: ensure the airway is protected/gag reflex is present (facial CPAP only) and GCS > 8

NO
CPAP not appropriate therapy
- Review resuscitation status and document
- Consider referral to ITU team for advice/ invasive ventilation if for attempted resuscitation
- Consider referral to respiratory team for NIV
- Consider use of opiates if DNAR decision made

YES ← **Criteria for CPAP still met?**

Medical staff
- Ensure patient and family are aware of treatment plans and that the patient agrees to the therapy if able
- **Prescribe CPAP** documenting goals: oxygen saturations, inspired oxygen concentration and cm of PEEP (available in 5 cm, 7.5 cm and 10 cm)
- Establish if the CPAP therapy will need to be intermittent or continuous: **Continuous CPAP therapy is only needed if oxygen saturations cannot be maintained > or equal to 93% on 60% fixed performance oxygen or more**
- Also review: iv access, 12-lead ECG, full bloods, iv fluids, fluid balance and nutritional status
- Ensure physiotherapy referral made
- Review drug chart: e.g. oral drugs may need to be given ng/iv, prescribe 2–4 hourly saline nebulisers
- Review nutritional requirements: if the patient is on continuous CPAP and or NBM consider commencing enteral nutrition or TPN
- Ensure nasogastric tube in situ within 12 hours of commencing CPAP to prevent gastric distension
- Document management plan if CPAP fails in medical notes: is this the ceiling intervention or is the patient appropriate for invasive/non-invasive ventilation? Consult the ITU team if felt appropriate
- Document resuscitation status

Nursing staff
Prepare the patient
- Commence at least hourly manual observation of TPR, BP, inspired oxygen % and oxygen saturations
- Ensure patient is nursed in the high dependency area of the ward unless isolated
- Ensure patient has a urinary catheter in situ unless contraindicated
- Commence hourly fluid balance monitoring
- Check blood sugar at least 6 hourly if LOC reduced/ NBM/TPN
- Unless contraindicated: sit the patient upright, administer 2–4 hourly nebuliser therapies, analgesia, oral fluids, perform mouth care, place Tegasorb on bridge of nose (if for facial CPAP) and ensure an appropriate pressure relieving mattress and electronic bed-frame is in use if available
- Aspirate any nasogastic tube 2–4 hourly to prevent gastric distension
- Consider use of 1:1 nursing depending on patient acuity and location

Prepare the environment
- Ensure a size G oxygen cylinder and Venturi or tracheostomy mask and nebuliser is at the bedside for delivery of oxygen/nebuliser therapy whenever CPAP is removed
- Ensure bedside suction is functioning (normal pressure 125 mmHg) plus a Yankauer sucker and suction catheters are available
- Get a CPAP generator, oxygen analyser, pressure gauge, and oxygen saturation monitor and disposable circuit

Figure 5.4 Example of CPAP algorithm. With kind permission from Royal Free Hampstead NHS Trust. ABG, arterial blood gases; CXR, chest radiograph; LOC, level of consciousness; GCS, Glasgow Coma Scale; ITU, intensive care unit; NIV, non-invasive ventilation; DNAR, do not attempt resuscitation; PEEP, positive end-expiratory pressure; iv, intravenous; ECG, electrocardiogram; ng, nasogastric; NBM, nil by mouth; TPN, total parenteral nutrition; TPR, termperature, pulse respiration; BP, blood pressure.

CPAP and how on-going monitoring should be provided. It will also describe how emergency situations should be dealt with and where CPAP can safely be offered in the individual healthcare environment.

A CPAP algorithm (Figure 5.4) to aid clinical decision making will enable the provision of safe and effective practice with a clear indication of which healthcare professionals will carry the responsibility for the provision of CPAP.

A prescription chart indicating both the levels of required therapy and how much the patient has received, will ensure that therapy is optimised.

Service requirements

When instituting a service to deliver CPAP, the following issues should be considered:

- Service location
- Staff skill mix
- Competencies
- Number and location of staff involved
- Rolling teaching programme
- Clinical supervision

The location of the service must be in a setting which has staff regularly trained to manage patients using CPAP. This will require a regular programme of training to support this which will ensure the competency of staff to make clinical decisions and to troubleshoot where patients are not responding to treatment. A service of this nature will require a minimum number of staff to be available over all shifts in order to ensure that all patients receive safe and effective care. In addition, clinical supervision may provide a practical way of developing problem-solving skills in junior staff.

Case study 5.1   CPAP for the treatment of sputum retention post cardiothoracic surgery

Andrew is a 48-year-old dentist who has had a coronary artery bypass graft to three coronary arteries yesterday. He is overweight and has a history of smoking. He went to the ICU after his surgery where he remained overnight. He was extubated at 0800 hours this morning when his arterial blood gases on FiO_2 60% via a Venturi mask were:

Case study 5.1   (Continued)

pH	7.33
$PaCO_2$	4.5
PaO_2	9.5

He was transferred to the high dependency unit. Two hours later Andrew complained of pain over his sternal wound and was not able to perform his breathing exercises or chest clearance with the physiotherapist. On chest X-ray, collapse of both lower lobes was noted and he had pyrexia at 38 °C. His latest arterial blood gases on 60% oxygen are:

pH	7.33
$PaCO_2$	4.5
PaO_2	7.5

Andrew is assessed by an anaesthetist and a decision made to start high-flow CPAP with oxygen at 60% and a PEEP pressure of 10 cmH$_2$O. Physiologically this will correct his functional residual capacity which will have been reduced because he is overweight and has undergone surgery, it will correct his hypoxaemia and provide positive expiratory pressure which will maximise oxygenation by keeping the alveoli open for longer during expiration allowing longer time for gaseous exchange. Arterial blood gases immediately after commencing CPAP are taken:

pH	7.33
$PaCO_2$	4.5
PaO_2	10.02

The CPAP regimen for Andrew is that he will use it continuously for the next 4 hours with short breaks of 5 minutes every hour for oral care and hydration. He is monitored every half an hour by the high dependency nurse and observations of respiratory rate, SpO$_2$, heart rate, blood pressure, breathing pattern, comfort, sputum colour and volume. He also receives physiotherapy to aid sputum clearance, improve oxygenation and begin mobilising gently. After 4 hours his arterial blood gases are repeated:

pH	7.33
$PaCO_2$	4.5
PaO_2	11.02

A decision is now taken to wean Andrew off the CPAP by decreasing its use to 30 minutes every 2 hours. Andrew is also encouraged to drink fluids and take regular saline nebulisers to encourage sputum clearance. Monitoring is continued as described earlier and Andrew takes a short walk up and down the high dependency unit in the afternoon with the physiotherapist.

Overnight Andrew uses the CPAP until he settles for the night. A decision not to continue with CPAP during the night is taken as his SpO$_2$ is now 95–96% on 60% via a Venturi mask. The following morning Andrew is able to expectorate mucoid green sputum independently and his SpO$_2$ is now 95% on 40% oxygen. CPAP is not re-commenced and Andrew's recovery is uneventful. He is discharged 6 days following surgery.

Case study 5.2 CPAP for the treatment of rib fractures after a road traffic accident

Harold is a 78-year-old man and was crossing the road on a zebra crossing when he was knocked down by a speeding car. He was admitted to hospital via the emergency department, with a broken right femur and eight rib fractures on the right. He was alert and orientated. He was a smoker and has been admitted to hospital because of his breathing on one occasion. His SpO_2 in the emergency department is 93% on room air and his chest X-ray shows multiple rib fractures on the right and a right pneumothorax; he has a chest drain inserted on the right in the emergency department which drains haemoserous fluid and partially inflates the right lung.

Harold is transferred to the respiratory ward and has observations of respiratory rate, heart rate, SpO_2 and breathing pattern every 30 minutes. Two hours after being admitted to the respiratory ward, Harold is mildly confused: he is not complaining of any pain as long as he does not attempt to move. He has received physiotherapy but has not been able to perform any breathing exercises or coughing because it is too painful. He is transferred to a high dependency unit and given an epidural for pain relief to enable him to move cough and expectorate. A repeat chest X-ray shows increased shadowing throughout the right lung. The chest drain is swinging and bubbling and the lung has remained inflated. Arterial blood gases on 60% are as follows:

pH	7.30
$PaCO_2$	7.6
PaO_2	8.3
SpO_2	90%

A decision is taken to give CPAP using a PEEP valve of 7.5 cmH_2O with 60% oxygen using a regimen of 50 minutes on CPAP followed by 10 minutes using oxygen via a Venturi mask at 60%, to enable regular sputum clearance, nebulisers, oral hydration and movement about the bed area. This decision is taken as although Harold has some history of COPD, it is known that he is not hypercapnic; as a result CPAP is the treatment of choice to provide adequate oxygenation. Harold receives physiotherapy four times over the course of the day and starts to expectorate independently. He appears more orientated and his SpO_2 on 60% oxygen via a Venturi mask is now 93%. His arterial blood gases are now:

pH	7.33
$PaCO_2$	6.5
PaO_2	10.32

Both his PaO_2 and $PaCO_2$ have started to correct as he has been able to start expectorating. He receives CPAP throughout the night following the regimen described above. Over the course of the following day, Harold receives CPAP with 50% oxygen for alternate hours together with three sessions of physiotherapy. By the afternoon his SpO_2 is 96% on 50% oxygen via a Venturi mask and CPAP therapy is stopped.

Over the course of the next few days Harold expectorates independently and his chest X-ray clears. His chest drain is removed and he receives regular ongoing physiotherapy to aid in the rehabilitation of his fracture femur.

CPAP for the treatment of obstructive sleep apnoea/hypopnoea syndrome

Principles of treatment

CPAP, generated by a small, portable electrically powered compressor, is used in the treatment of obstructive sleep apnoea/hypopnoea syndrome (OSAHS) and delivers pressure at a continuous level throughout the respiratory cycle. Patients with OSAHS need to use CPAP in order to maintain an open airway during sleep which obviates the effects of airway obstruction, described later. Oxygen can be entrained via the mask or a T piece, but many patients do not need additional oxygen.

Prevalence of sleep-related breathing disorders

Sleep disorders in general prevent a person from getting restful sleep, and as a result can cause daytime sleepiness and psychological and physical dysfunction. There are approximately eight types of sleep disorder, the most common being:

- Insomnia
- Sleep apnoea
- Restless leg syndrome
- Narcolepsy

The reported prevalence of OSAHS varies according to the source of the information. Young & Finn (1998) found a prevalence of 4% in middle-aged men and 2% in middle-aged women, which equates to approximately 650 000 people with the condition in the UK. These figures are corroborated by Fogel et al. (2004) who found that OSAHS affected 2–4% of middle-aged men and women in the USA. The Sleep Apnoea Trust estimates that 80 000 people in the UK have OSAHS, most of whom are male and overweight (www.sleep-apnoea-trust.org). The Sleep Alliance in its 'Sleep SOS Report' (2005) estimated that 1–2% of men, and fewer than half that number of women have OSAHS. This equates to 300 000 men and 80 000 women who have OSAHS in the UK. However, as Young et al. (1997) reported, it is estimated that many patients go undiagnosed (93% of women and 82% of men).

OSAHS is caused by collapse of the upper airway during sleep. This leads to a requirement for increased effort to overcome the obstruction with consequent arousal from deep sleep to allow normal muscle tone to be established. These obstructions are classified either as apnoeas, which allow no airflow for 10 seconds, or hypopnoeas, which cause hypoventilation resulting in reduced airflow by 50% over a 10-second period. The severity of OSAHS is determined by the apnoea/hypopnoea index (AHI) on polysomnography and indicates the number of apnoea or hypopnoeas occurring overnight per hour. OSAHS is defined as mild (AHI 5–14/h), moderate (AHI 15–30/h) or severe (AHI >30/h).

The primary symptoms of OSAHS are daytime somnolence and sleep disturbance or snoring, as listed below, but the other effects should be noted, and overall a patient's quality of life may be poor as a result. In addition, partners may also be sleep deprived because of the patient's OSAHS and relationships may be adversely affected. The insidious nature of the condition contributes to difficulties in its treatment, particularly in relation to acceptance of therapies such as CPAP, as patients may have little appreciation of how much they are affected by the condition until they are successfully treated.

The symptoms of sleep apnoea include (Schlosshan & Elliott, 2004):

- Snoring
- Apnoea and nocturnal choking
- Daytime hypersomnolence
- Increased risk of car accidents
- Impaired concentration
- Irritability
- Low mood
- Loss of libido
- Nightmares
- Reduced quality of life
- Personality change
- Interference with quality of personal relationships

Burden of OSAHS

Possible impacts of OSAHS on health include cardiovascular mortality and morbidity, hypertension, and a possible role in motor vehicle accidents. Peker et al. (2002) found that in a cohort of previously healthy middle-aged men with incompletely treated OSAHS there was marked increase in cardiovascular disease during a 7-year follow-up period. Peker et al. (2006) found that coronary heart disease was confirmed in 24.6% of 65 incompletely treated patients compared with 3.9% of efficiently treated subjects concluding that efficient treatment of OSAHS reduced the risk of coronary heart disease. Rauscher et al. (1992) found that

40% of patients with resistant hypertension had detectable OSAHS while Pepperell et al. (2002) found that 40% of patients with OSAHS were hypertensive. George (2001) showed a decrease in road accidents following the treatment of sleep apnoea with CPAP therapy. Douglas and George (2002) quantified the potential savings by treating 500 patients with CPAP as £1.3 million.

Patients with chronic lung disease may have significant arterial oxygen desaturation during the rapid eye movement (REM) phase of sleep when chest wall movement is decreased, which therefore decreases tidal and minute volume. In addition, many patients with chronic lung disease also experience hypoventilation during sleep. This compounds arterial oxygen desaturation and may contribute to the development of complications such as pulmonary hypertension, cardiac dysrhythmias and cognitive impairment (Ryan, 2005). It is therefore imperative that sleep apnoea/hypoventilation is detected in these patients and treated accordingly.

Assessment of sleep disorders

A preliminary screening questionnaire such as the Epworth sleepiness scale (Figure 5.5) may be used to detect whether a patient requires further investigation (Johns, 1991).

The 6-point scale is a questionnaire with a maximum score of 24, which enables an estimation to be made of the subjective perception of sleepiness. Both the patient and their partner should complete it as patients may underestimate their levels of somnolence. Scores range from normal subjective daytime sleepiness (<11), mild 11–14, moderate 15–18 or severe >18. Those with an Epworth sleepiness scale score of greater than 10 should be referred for further investigation of their sleep apnoea.

Sleep studies include a range of technologies that are used to study and diagnose a variety of sleep-breathing problems, including sleep disruption from airway obstruction and nocturnal ventilatory failure as a result of primary pulmonary disease, e.g. chronic obstructive pulmonary disease (COPD), kyphoscoliosis, thoracoplasty. The tests involve monitoring the patient while asleep and making measurements including chest wall movement, airflow through the nose and mouth, oxygen levels in the blood, arousal rates (e.g. increase in pulse rate), sleep staging and monitoring of body position. The key outcome measures of sleep-disordered breathing are daytime measures of sleepiness and blood gas levels (Figures 5.6 and 5.7).

Sleep studies fall into five different types:

The Epworth Sleepiness Scale

Name: _____

Today's date: _____ Your age (years): _____

Your sex (male = M; female = F): _____

How likely are you to doze off or fall asleep in the following situations, in contrast to feeling just tired? This refers to your usual way of life in recent times. Even if you have not done some of these things recently try to work out how they would have affected you. Use the following scale to choose the *most appropriate number* for each situation:

    0 = would *never* doze
    1 = *slight* chance of dozing
    2 = *moderate* change of dozing
    3 = *high* chance of dozing

Situation	Chance of dozing
Sitting and reading	_____
Watching TV	_____
Sitting, inactive in a public place (e.g. a theater or a meeting)	_____
As a passenger in a car for an hour without a break	_____
Lying down to rest in the afternoon when circumstances permit	_____
Sitting and talking to someone	_____
Sitting quietly after a lunch without alcohol	_____
In a car, while stopped for a few minutes in the traffic	_____

Thank you for your cooperation

Figure 5.5 Epworth sleepiness scale. With kind permission from American Academy of Sleep Medicine.

- Simple pulse oximetry and/or snoring detection.
- Overnight video oximetry – not used generally in view of video requirement.
- Overnight multi-channel sleep study using fewer than five channels (airflow, oximetry, pulse, chest movement, snore detection, movement, position etc) or greater than five channels (with abdominal movement, airway pressure measurement, electromyography (EMG)). This equipment is designed for home or hospital use.
- Transcutaneous blood gas monitoring – which measures carbon dioxide; it is necessary to monitor patients with overnight hypoventilation and those requiring home ventilation. Use of this equipment will need an overnight hospital stay.
- Full polysomnography (PSG) which includes multi-channel testing plus sleep staging. A PSG typically involves an electroencephalogram (EEG), segmental tibialis electromyogram, electro-oculogram, respiratory airflow, thoraco-abdominal movement, oxygen saturation

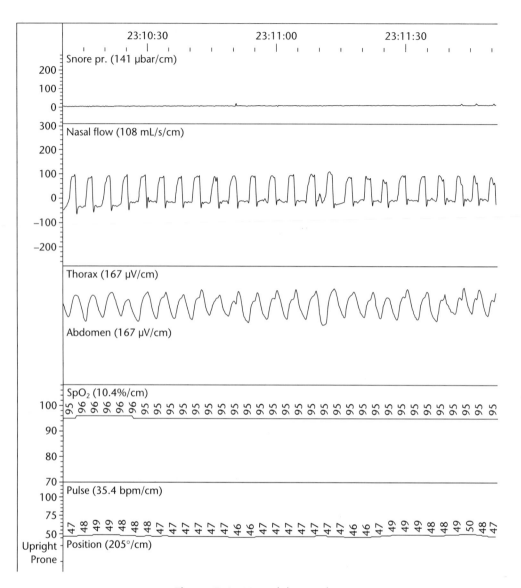

Figure 5.6 Normal sleep study.

tracings, electrocardiogram, body position and snoring. These studies should be used to diagnose sleep disturbance in selected complex cases only: its clinical value in establishing a diagnosis in all patients with daytime somnolence has not been confirmed. In addition, it requires an overnight hospital stay with technical support to set it up, monitoring throughout the night and specialist interpretation of the results.

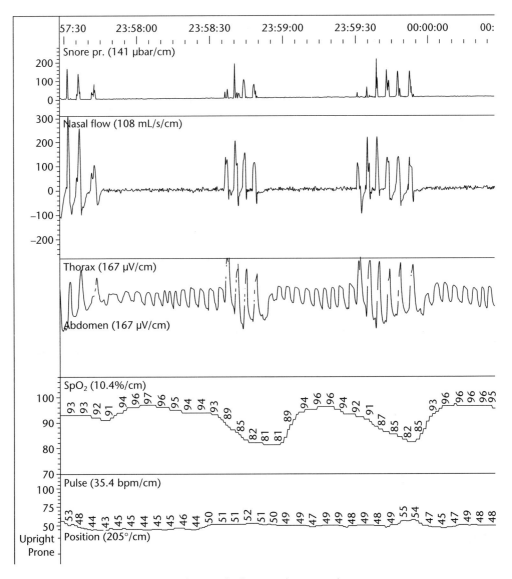

Figure 5.7 Sleep study showing obstructive sleep apnoea.

Treatment for sleep apnoea

Life-style changes

Obesity is a major risk factor for OSAHS with two-thirds of patients with OSAHS being obese (>120% of ideal body weight). Weight loss should therefore be advised for the overweight patient although there is a poor correlation with loss of weight and clinical outcome (Smith et al., 1985).

Life-style changes aiming to promote good sleep hygiene should be encouraged and may include avoiding alcohol in the evening and not taking sedatives or sleeping tablets, as each of these promote relaxation of the upper airway and hence increase sleep apnoea. Smoking cessation should also be encouraged as smoking has been linked to OSAHS (Jennum & Sjol, 1992). Patients should be advised to stop smoking in conjunction with dietary control to minimise the potential side effect of weight gain on stopping smoking. In addition, patients may find a weight loss programme easier to adhere to if their OSAHS is treated simultaneously with CPAP, as this will confer benefits which will encourage greater activity and hence speedier weight loss. The National Institute for Health and Clinical Excellence (NICE) guidelines (NICE, 2008) recommend that CPAP should be used for those with moderate to severely symptomatic OSAHS but only in those who are mildly symptomatic after life-style changes have been tried first.

Equipment

CPAP involves the use of a small electrically driven pump connected via tubing to a nasal mask which is worn throughout the night, during sleep (Figure 5.8). Patients with OSAHS do not usually require oxygen except in the presence of obesity hypoventilation syndrome. Such patients may additionally have Type II respiratory failure as a complication of their sleep apnoea. In these cases, low levels of oxygen (usually no more then 2–3 l/min) may be required and can be delivered at home via an oxygen concentrator. It is connected to the CPAP circuit using either a T piece or a port on the CPAP mask. Where it proves difficult to maintain a good seal, it may be necessary to use a face mask in preference to a nasal mask for the delivery of the CPAP. Patients who are prescribed the use of a CPAP machine at home must be capable of using it safely and independently and be instructed in the care of the machine and the circuit to optimise its use and effectiveness (see below).

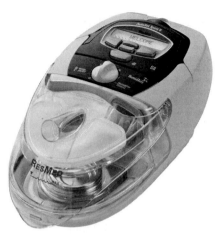

Figure 5.8 CPAP for the treatment of obstructive sleep apnoea. With kind permission from Resmed.

CPAP machines consist of two types of machine: fixed pressure and auto-titrating machines. Fixed pressure CPAP machines deliver a pressure constantly throughout the night and require that this pre-set pressure is initially determined by a sleep study. Auto-titrating CPAP machines alter their pressure according to the level of obstruction and can be used both as a treatment and as a tool to determine the pressure settings required for treatment. The idea supporting the use of an auto-titrating machine is that it is more comfortable with less mask leak and fewer side effects as a result of lower flows (Meurice et al., 1996). However, some anecdotal evidence suggests that changes in pressure may, in itself, lead to disturbance of sleep.

Side effects of CPAP

The following side effects may occur as a result of using CPAP:

- Rhinitis
- Sinusitis
- Epistaxis
- Glabellar (nasal bridge) sores
- Abdominal bloating

Adherence with CPAP

Reasons for non-adherence with CPAP include:

- Discomfort
- Poor mask fit
- Glabellar (nasal bridge) sores
- Pressure intolerance
- Nasal dryness, irritation or bleeding
- Noise
- Claustrophobia

Regular follow-up will help to alleviate many of the above issues and patients may benefit from the use of heated humidification or a cortico-steroid nasal spray in the presence of rhinitis or dryness of the nose. Where mask leak is a problem it may be necessary to re-fit the mask, possibly trying the use of either a chin strap or a full face mask as an alternative.

Psychological impact on patients and their families

Adequate discussion and information must be given to patients and their relatives prior to beginning treatment with CPAP to promote its use and encourage adherence. CPAP therapy requires commitment on behalf of the patient and its psychological impact should not be over-looked. Scores for anxiety and depression have been shown to improve significantly following treatment in mild and severe cases of OSAHS (NHMRC, 2000). Patients have reported feeling stigmatised by needing to use this type of equipment at home and being afraid that they will scare children and grandchildren (Mikelsons et al., 2006). Compliance with this type of therapy has, in some cases, been reported to be as low as 40% but benefits can produce valuable changes in quality of life, ability to work and in personal relationships and every effort should be made to promote use. More recently, techniques such as cognitive behaviour therapy, provided at the beginning of therapy, have shown to produce a marked improvement in compliance with CPAP of up to 148% (Richards & Bartlett, 2007).

Employment/driving

The effects of OSAHS may be profound in terms of interference with ability to perform a job. It may interfere with the ability to stay awake while working or talking on the phone or may make keeping a job impossible because of depression, irritability or learning and memory difficulties.

In terms of driving, the prevalence of OSAHS is known to be high among lorry drivers (Stoohs et al., 1995). When a person is diagnosed with OSAHS they must be informed in writing and verbally that it is their responsibility to inform the Driver and Vehicle Licensing Authority (DVLA) of the diagnosis. However, as long a patient complies with treatment there should be no issue about retaining their licence. In the case of heavy goods vehicle drivers this must be confirmed by a specialist in sleep disorders.

Patient information

The following information should be given to patients at diagnosis of OSAHS:

- Causes of sleep apnoea
- Who gets it and why
- Symptoms of sleep apnoea
- The risks of untreated sleep apnoea
- Use and care of CPAP equipment, its side effects, mask care and follow-up
- Contact telephone numbers
- Driving and informing the DVLA

For an example of a patient information sheet for OSAHS, see Chapter 6.

Other forms of treatment

Dental devices

Dental devices which produce an anterior displacement of the mandible such as mandibular advancement splints are designed to change the patency of the upper airway and thus increase its diameter. There is evidence supporting their use in mild cases of OSAHS but at present evidence is lacking for in their use in severe cases (Scottish Intercollegiate Guidelines Network (SIGN), 2003).

Surgical interventions

Surgical interventions such as uvulopalatopharyngoplasty (UPPP) in the treatment of OSAHS are not recommended (SIGN, 2003).

Drug therapy

Drug therapy to increase ventilatory drive or suppress REM sleep are rarely used in practice in view of the side effects (Ryan, 2005) and are not recommended as first-line treatment for OSAHS (SIGN, 2003).

Case study 5.3   CPAP for treatment of obstructive sleep apnoea

Larry is a 45-year-old long-distance lorry driver. He is obese and suffers from hypertension. He is attending the sleep clinic because his wife had complained of his snoring – it is keeping her awake for much of the night. In addition she has noticed that Larry stops breathing frequently and she is afraid that he may not start breathing again when this happens. Larry falls asleep in front of the television, cannot stay awake during conversations and even falls asleep while waiting to see the doctor in clinic. He describes feeling not refreshed by sleep, being short tempered and lacking in libido. He does not have any energy to participate in any activities outside the home except for trips to the pub in the evening which he feels may help him sleep. He also tries to alleviate his poor sleep by taking sleeping tablets. Larry realises that he should do more to lose weight but lacks motivation and feels low in mood much of the time. Larry was screened using the Epworth scale to determine if he has sleep apnoea. He scored 17 on the scale indicating that he does have sleep apnoea. He was underwent an overnight sleep study at home, which showed he had an AHI of 29 with the lowest saturation at 80%. The DVLA was informed and Larry had to stop working while he waited for his CPAP machine to be supplied. When he was supplied the CPAP, he attempted to use it but struggled until he attended the sleep clinic for a re-fitting of the mask and headgear. He eventually managed to complete a whole night on the machine and on waking found he was refreshed by his sleep and that his wife was not complaining of being kept awake all night. Once Larry was established on CPAP, the DVLA was informed that he was being treated successfully and he resumed working as a lorry driver.

Case study 5.4   Obesity hypoventilation syndrome

Sam is a 68-year-old man with obesity, hypertension and Type 2 diabetes. He attended at his outpatient appointment complaining of hypersomnolence, irritability and low mood. He reports that others have complained that he snores during sleep. His Epworth score was 20 and a sleep study identified that he has an AHI of 30/h with a fall in saturation down to 85% during sleep. He was diagnosed as having obesity hypoventilation syndrome. He was prescribed a CPAP machine set to 8 cmH$_2$O from a low-flow machine without added oxygen. At a follow-up appointment in the outpatient clinic 6 weeks later, he presented with shortness of breath on minimal exertion and difficulty in completing his activities of daily living. He was cyanosed and his SpO$_2$ was 74% on room air. His arterial blood gases on room air were found to be the following:

pH	7.4
PaCO$_2$	6.29
PaO$_2$	4.94

On 1 litre of oxygen, his repeat arterial blood gases were:

pH	7.36
PaCO$_2$	6.79
PaO$_2$	6.85

As his hypoxaemia was not corrected and his hypercapnia was worsened, using 1 litre of oxygen, the decision was taken to admit Sam for further treatment. He received NIV using a bi-level ventilator set to an inspiratory positive airway pressure (IPAP) of 20 and an expiratory positive airway pressure (EPAP) of 4 with 2 litres of oxygen, to correct his arterial blood gases and decrease his work of breathing. His arterial blood gases on NIV were:

pH	7.36
PaCO$_2$	5.9
PaO$_2$	8.5

When Sam was not on the ventilator, oxygen was given at 2 litres via nasal cannulae as this was the most comfortable form of delivery for him. Sam remained on NIV for the next 4 days, during which time he was taught exercises to improve his exercise tolerance. Prior to discharge home his arterial blood gases on room air were:

pH	7.36
PaCO$_2$	6.00
PaO$_2$	8.35

Sam is continuing with his CPAP therapy without oxygen, as before. The use of NIV during this acute onset of respiratory failure corrected Sam's arterial blood gases so that he was able to return to using CPAP at home; however, in future it may be necessary to change his CPAP for NIV in order to provide adequate respiratory support in the presence of progressive respiratory failure. In addition a careful eye must be kept on Sam's requirement for additional long-term oxygen therapy so that it can be prescribed once it is required (PaO$_2$ < 7.3).

Case study 5.5   CPAP for the treatment of cardiogenic pulmonary oedema

Amita is a 78-year-old woman with a history of silent myocardial infarction and angina for the past 5 years. She presented to the emergency department with a 3-day history of worsening shortness of breath at rest (Medical Research Council (MRC) grade 5), ankle oedema and an SpO_2 of 84%. She is usually limited in her activities of daily living by her breathlessness, cannot manage the stairs at home and does not go out. She was transferred to the coronary care unit (CCU) for monitoring of her cardiac and vital signs. She and her family have discussed her management at the end of her life and do not want any interventions which would prolong the inevitable, but do want her to be actively cared for. On transferring to CCU, Amita's blood pressure (BP) is 160/90 mmHg, central venous pressure is 20 cmH_2O, arterial blood gases: pH 7.33, $PaCO_2$ 5.6, PaO_2 6.5, chest X-ray shows butterfly shadowing radiating from both central hila. She is given 60% oxygen via a Venturi mask which improves her PaO_2 to 7.5. She is also given amiodarone, diuretics and is on controlled fluid intake. She remains very breathless at rest and a decision is made to treat her with CPAP at 7.5 cmH_2O via a face mask with 60% oxygen. Her arterial blood gases on CPAP are:

pH	7.34
$PaCO_2$	5.3
PaO_2	9.5

She remains on CPAP for 2 hours continuously and then receives it following a regimen of 1 hour on CPAP, followed by a 30-minute break continued throughout the next 24 hours. The following day Amita has returned to her previous levels of breathlessness (MRC 3), CPAP is stopped and she starts to mobilise gently around the ward.

References

American Association of Respiratory Care (1993) Clinical Practice Guideline Respiratory Care. Use of positive pressure adjuncts to bronchial hygiene therapy. *Respiratory Care*, **38**, 516–521.

Bellone, A., Monari, A., Cortellaro, F., Vettorello, M., Arlati, S. & Coen, D. (2004) Myocardial infarction rate in acute pulmonary edema: non-invasive pressure support ventilation versus continuous positive airway pressure. *Critical Care Medicine*, **32**, 1860–1865.

Bellone, A., Vettorello, M., Monari, A., Cortellaro, F. & Coen, D. (2005) Non-invasive pressure support ventilation vs. continuous positive airway. pressure in acute hypercapnic pulmonary edema. *Intensive Care Medicine*, **31**, 807–11.

Bersten, A.D., Holt, A.W., Vedig, A.E., Skowronski, G.A. & Baggoley, C.J. (1991) Treatment of severe cardiogenic pulmonary oedema with continuous positive airway pressure delivery by face mask. *New England Journal of Medicine*, **325**, 1825–1830.

Bolliger, C.T. & Van Eeden, S.F. (1990) Treatment of multiple rib fractures. Randomised controlled trial comparing ventilatory with nonventilatory management. *Chest*, **97**, 943–948.

British Thoracic Society Standards of Care Committee (2002) British Thoracic Society Guideline. Non-invasive ventilation in acute respiratory care. *Thorax*, **57**, 192–211.

Crane, S.D., Elliott, M.W., Gilligan, P., Richards, K. & Gray, A.J. (2004) Randomised controlled comparison of continuous positive airways pressure, bilevel non-invasive ventilation, and standard treatment in emergency department patients with acute cardiogenic pulmonary oedema. *Emergency Medicine Journal*, **21**, 155–161.

Douglas, N.J. & George, C.F.P. (2002) Treating sleep apnoea is cost effective. *Thorax*, **57**, 93.

Downs, J.B. (2003) Has oxygen administration delayed appropriate respiratory care? Fallacies regarding oxygen therapy. *Respiratory Care*, **48**, 611–620.

Fogel, R.B., Malhotra, A. & White, D.P. (2004) Sleep × 2, pathophysiology of obstructive sleep apnoea/hypopnoea syndrome. *Thorax*, **59**, 159–163.

George, C.F. (2001) Sleep × 5, Driving and automobile crashes in patients with obstructive sleep apnoea/hypopnoea syndrome. *Thorax*, **59**, 804–807.

Jennum, P. & Sjol, A. (1992) Epidemiology of snoring and obstructive sleep apnoea in a Danish population, age 30–60. *Journal of Sleep Research*, **1**, 240–244.

Johns, M.W. (1991) A new method for measuring daytime sleepiness: the Epworth sleepiness scale. *Sleep*, **14**, 540–545.

Lin M, Yang, Y.F., Chiang, H.T., Chang, M.S., Chiang, B.N. & Cheitlin, M.D. (1995) Reappraisal of CPAP therapy in acute pulmonary oedema: short-term results and long-term follow up. *Chest*, **107**, 1379–1386.

Lindner, K.H., Lotz, P. & Ahnefeld, F.W. (1987) Continuous positive airway pressure effect on functional residual capacity, vital capacity and its subdivisions. *Chest*, **92**, 66–70.

Martin-Bermudez, R.J., Rodriguez-Portal, J.A., Garcia-Garmendia, J.L., Garcia-Diaz, E., Montano-Diaz, M., Soto-Espinosa, B., Murillo-Cabezas, F. & Muniz-Grijalvo, O. (2002) Non-invasive ventilation in cardiogenic pulmonary edema. Preliminary results of a randomized trial. *Intensive Care Medicine*, **28**, S68.

Mehta, S., Jay, G.D., Woolard, R.H., Hipona, R.A., Connolly, E.M., Cimini, D.M., Drinkwine, J.H. & Hill, N.S. (1997) Randomized, prospective trial of bilevel versus continuous positive airway pressure in acute pulmonary edema. *Critical Care Medicine*, **25**, 620–628.

Meurice, J.C., Marc, I. & Series, F. (1996) Efficacy of auto-CPAP in the treatment of obstructive sleep apnoea/hypopnoea syndrome. *American Journal of Respiratory Critical Care Medicine*, **153**, 794–798.

Mikelsons, C., Muncey, T. & Wedzicha, J.A. (2006) Experience of chronic obstructive pulmonary disease patients using home non-invasive ventilation. *Thorax*, **61** (Suppl 2), ii57–ii133 (P182).

National Health and Medical Research Council (2000) *Effectiveness of Nasal Continuous Positive Airway Pressure in Obstructive Sleep Apnoea in Adults*. Canberra: The Council. Available at: http://www.nhmrc.gov.au/publications/synopses/hpr21syn.htm (accessed 17 May 2008).

National Institute for Health and Clinical Excellence (NICE) (2008) Continuous positive airway pressure for the treatment of obstructive sleep apnoea/hypopnoea syndrome. Technical appraisal 139. NICE, London. Available at: www.nice.org.uk/ta139 (accessed 17 May 2008).

Park, M., Lorenzi-Filho, G., Feltrim, M.I., Viecili, P.R., Sangean, M.C., Volpe, M., Leite, P.F. & Mansur, A.J. (2001) Oxygen therapy, continuous positive airway pressure, or noninvasive bilevel positive pressure ventilation in the treatment of acute cardiogenic pulmonary edema. *Arquivos Brasileiros de Cardiologia*, **76**, 221–230.

Park, M., Sangean, M.C., Volpe M, S., Feltrim, M.I., Nozawa, E., Leite, P.F., Passos Amato, M.B. & Lorenzi-Filho G. (2004) Randomized, prospective trial of oxygen, continuous positive airway pressure, and bilevel positive airway pressure by face mask in acute cardiogenic pulmonary edema. *Critical Care Medicine*, **32**, 2407–2415.

Peker, Y., Hedner, J., Norum, J., Kraiczi, H. & Carlson, J. (2002) Increased incidence of cardiovascular disease in obstructive sleep apnoea. *American Journal of Respiratory and Critical Care Medicine*, **166**, 159–165.

Peker, Y., Carlson, J. & Hedner, J. (2006) Increased incidence of coronary artery disease in sleep apnoea: a long-term follow up. *European Respiratory Journal*, **28**, 596–602.

Pepperell, J.C., Ramdassingh-Dow, S., Crosthwaite, N., Mullins, R., Jenkinson, C., Stradling, J.R. & Davies, R.J. (2002) Ambulatory blood pressure after therapeutic and subtherapeutic nasal continuous positive airway pressure for obstructive sleep apnoea: a randomised parallel trial. *Lancet*, **359**, 204–210.

Pryor, J.A. & Prasad, S.A. (eds) (2002) *Physiotherapy for Respiratory and Cardiac Problems*, 3rd ed. Churchill Livingstone, Edinburgh.

Rauscher, H., Popp, W. & Zwick, H. (1992) Systemic hypertension in snorers with and without sleep apnoea. *Chest*, **102**, 367–371.

Richards, D. & Bartlett, D. (2007). Increased adherence to CPAP with a group cognitive behavioral treatment intervention: a randomized trial. *Journal of Sleep*, **30**, 635–640.

Ryan, C.F. (2005) Sleep × 9, An approach to treatment of obstructive sleep apnoea/hypopnoea syndrome including upper airway surgery. *Thorax*, **60**, 595–604.

Schlosshan, D. & Elliott, M.W. (2004) Sleep × 3, Clinical presentation and diagnosis of the obstructive sleep apnoea/hypopnoea syndrome. *Thorax*, **59**, 347–352.

Scottish Intercollegiate Guidelines Network (2003) Management of obstructive sleep apnoea/hypopnoea syndrome in adults. A national clinical guideline. Scottish Intercollegiate Guidelines Network, Edinburgh.

Sleep Alliance (2005) Sleep SOS Report. Available at http://www.britishsnoring.co.uk/the_sleep_sos_report.php (accessed 17 May 2008).

Sleep Apnoea Trust. www.sleep-apnoea-trust.org

Smith, P.L., Gold, A.R., Meyers, D.A., Haponik, E.F. & Bleeker, E.R. (1985) Weight loss in mildly to moderately obese patients with obstructive sleep apnoea. *Annals of Internal Medicine*, **103**, 850–855.

Stock, M.C., Downs, J.B., Gauer, P.K., Alster, J.M. & Imrey, P.B. (1985) Prevention of postoperative pulmonary complications with CPAP, incentive spirometry and conservative therapy. *Chest*, **87**, 151–157.

Stoohs, R.A., Bingham, L.A., Itoi, A., Guilleminault, C. & Dement, W.C. (1995) Sleep and sleep-disordered breathing in commercial long-haul truck drivers. *Chest*, **107**, 1275–1282.

Winck, J.C., Azevedo, L.F., Costa-Pereira, A., Antonelli, M. & Wyatt, J.C. (2006) Efficacy and safety of non-invasive ventilation in the treatment of acute cardiogenic pulmonary edema – a systematic review and meta-analysis. *Critical Care*, **10**, 2–18.

Young, T. & Finn, L. (1998) Epidemiological insights into the public health burden of sleep disordered breathing: sex differences in survival among sleep clinic patients. *Thorax*, **53** (Suppl 3): S16–S19.

Young, T., Evans, L., Finn, L. & Palta M. (1997) Estimation of the clinically diagnosed proportion of sleep apnoea syndrome in middle aged men and women. *Sleep*, **20**, 705–706.

Chapter 6
SETTING UP RESPIRATORY SUPPORT SERVICES

This chapter will examine the practicalities of setting up services to provide:

- Acute non-invasive ventilation (NIV)
- Home NIV
- Home oxygen
- Home continuous positive airway pressure (CPAP) for sleep apnoea/hypopnoea syndrome

The setting up of respiratory support services requires careful planning, and once they are introduced they should be monitored to ensure that quality care is achieved and maintained. The principles for developing services for NIV, oxygen therapy and CPAP should be based on the key components of clinical governance (Figure 6.1), defined as:

'A framework through which NHS organisations are accountable for continuously improving the quality of their services and safeguarding high standards of care by creating an environment in which excellence in clinical care will flourish'

(Scally & Donaldson, 1998)

Clinical effectiveness is a key element of clinical governance and requires a sound knowledge of the evidence base which will underwrite competent practice (National Institute of Clinical Excellence (NICE), 2002; Royal College of Nursing, 2003). Patient safety is paramount and therefore a multi-disciplinary approach should be adopted so that skills that meet the patient's needs are available. Who within the team undertakes the different components of the services is not as important as individual staff members having the competencies in delivering these specialist services. As well as having the appropriate staff the service needs to be based on evidence-based clinical guidelines as

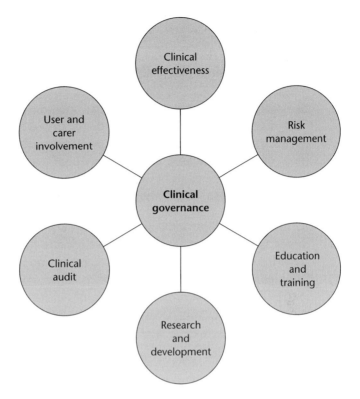

Figure 6.1 Key components of clinical governance.

discussed in previous chapters. Furthermore, advance planning prior to initiating a new or redesigning an existing service requires the following elements:

- Evidence-based protocols for clinical decision making.
- Staff education and competency.
- Clinical audit.
- Service development with a supporting business case that integrates with the commissioning framework.

To ensure both clinical effectiveness and the implementation of evidence-based practice, the necessity of continuing professional development is paramount as without this, clinicians will become out of date quickly as research which informs guidelines is ever changing.

Risk management is a statutory requirement and has implications in both the acute and home care settings. It involves the assessment of risk to patients, healthcare practitioners and the healthcare organisation. The aim is to minimise any identified risk factors so that wherever possible unnecessary risk is avoided. The process may involve risk registers, critical event audits and a robust complaints procedure.

Research and development forms an integral part of sound clinical effectiveness as this will provide the evidence base for practice and ensure that unanswered questions are addressed. All guidelines should now be evidence based and also highlight areas for future research. This is important as it influences funding for future research, thereby increasing clinical knowledge.

Clinical audit allows the structure review of clinical services against agreed performance standards. The Kennedy Report (2001) identified how information is essential for promoting standards and quality as it enables services to be planned, commissioned, implemented, managed and evaluated. This forms the basis of the audit cycle, which can be used to improve the quality of clinical care (Figure 6.2).

User and carer involvement is an important aspect in the planning and organisation of healthcare. The Royal College of Nursing (2003) identifies that patient involvement in decision making regarding healthcare is paramount, given that they are the experts in receiving health and social care; this is reflected in the *Expert Patients' Programme* (Department of Health, 2001).

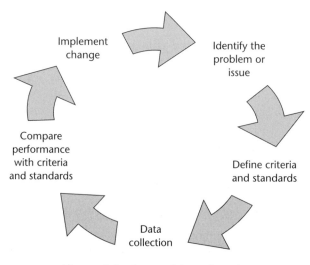

Figure 6.2   Stages of the audit cycle.

Non-invasive ventilation

The use of acute NIV in the context of service delivery is where the patient has intermittent NIV for the duration of an acute event, such as an exacerbation. It is likely that the patient will be critically ill during this phase and therefore there needs to be clear decision-making processes. For some patients the need for long-term NIV at home will become apparent either during their inpatient stay or at follow-up. However, it is important to recognise that not all patients requiring acute NIV will need to go on to receive long-term NIV. The principles of care are similar in both cases although the decision-making processes will be different.

Clinical decision making for acute NIV

A key consideration of the clinical decision-making process is the most appropriate environment, because if the patient is managed in an inappropriate environment there could be a significant risk to the patient. As this group consists of patients who are acutely ill they will require admission to a hospital which has an intensive care unit (ICU), as some patients initiated on NIV may need to be intubated if an adequate response to NIV is not achieved and if the multi-disciplinary team, along with the patient, feel this is an appropriate pathway of care. Within the acute hospital setting, there are then further considerations regarding the care setting in which the patient is being cared for. The following environments could be used:

- ICU
- High dependency unit (HDU)
- Respiratory ward
- General medical ward/medical assessment unit (MAU)

Plant et al. (2000) showed that patients can be safely managed on respiratory medical wards, although this is dependent on how acidotic the patient is and also the clinical expertise of the staff. It may be necessary to transfer patients who are critically ill with pH < 7.25 to level 3 (ICU) or level 2 (HDU) facilities (Department of Health, 2000). The decisions of when to transfer patients to different care environments will require clear clinical management plans determining:

- Patient selection including escalation of treatment and the ceiling of treatment (Figure 6.3).
- Resuscitation decisions and when end-of-life palliative care needs to be initiated.

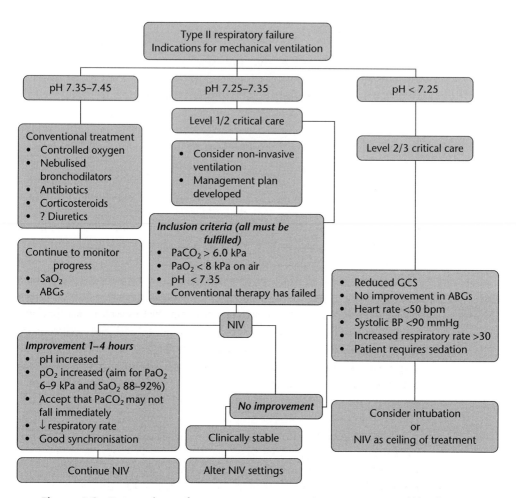

Figure 6.3   Patient selection for acute non-invasive ventilation. ABG, arterial blood gases; GCS, Glasgow Coma Scale; NIV, non-invasive ventilation; BP, blood pressure.

Clinical decision making based on clinical expertise should be guided by protocols. However, if there is deviation from the pathway within the protocol, a clear audit trail in relation to the decision-making processes should be available.

The environment in which the patient is cared for will be determined by the patient's clinical status. This will be guided by the arterial blood gas analysis, with particular emphasis on how acidotic the patient is (see Figure 6.3). However, the environment alone will not ensure quality patient outcomes. The multi-disciplinary team need to be skilled and competent in caring for critically ill patients using NIV. Furthermore, who is responsible for the various components of care needs to be determined. The following aspects need to be decided in relation to who is responsible for what:

- Assessment and suitability for treatment with NIV
- Prescribing treatment (type of machine and ventilator settings)
- Setting up patient on NIV
- Monitoring of patient (arterial blood gases, vital signs)
- Who is responsible for decision making overnight

Clinical decision making for home NIV

The use of home NIV in the context of service delivery is where the patient has NIV at home, usually overnight. Home NIV should only be given where a full assessment of the patient and their response to NIV has been evaluated in accordance with the evidence (Meecham-Jones et al., 1995). This may be done either at the end of an acute admission or after review during a stable period. In both cases, there must be a clear indication that the patient will benefit from its long-term use. Assessment should include arterial blood gases on and off NIV so that ventilator settings can be tailored to the individual patient. Furthermore, it must be ensured that the patient has the ability to manage the machine independently or that social support via a package of care is provided to assist the patient with using the NIV. Whether the patient self-manages or a carer provides support, the patient needs education and advice about its safe use. Figure 6.4 shows the patient selection criteria and pathway for home NIV.

Patients initiated on home NIV will be at an advanced stage of their disease, which will require additional support and treatment. Therefore, there need to be clear decision-making processes in place to ensure that this treatment is appropriate and end-of-life care considered and initiated when indicated, in line with recognised palliative care pathways such as the Liverpool Care Pathway for the Dying Patient (2004) and Gold Standard Framework (Department of Health, 2006).

Protocols and standards for NIV

One of the most important issues when deciding who is responsible for the various aspects of care is that the healthcare professionals are competent. To achieve this, healthcare professionals should have access to educational programmes covering key aspects of NIV care. In addition, there should be an opportunity for a period of supervised practice, allowing the healthcare professional to consolidate their education and to become competent. This will allow the theory–practice gap to be bridged and for the healthcare practitioner to encounter different challenging clinical situations under supervision. A competency assessment (Figure 6.5),

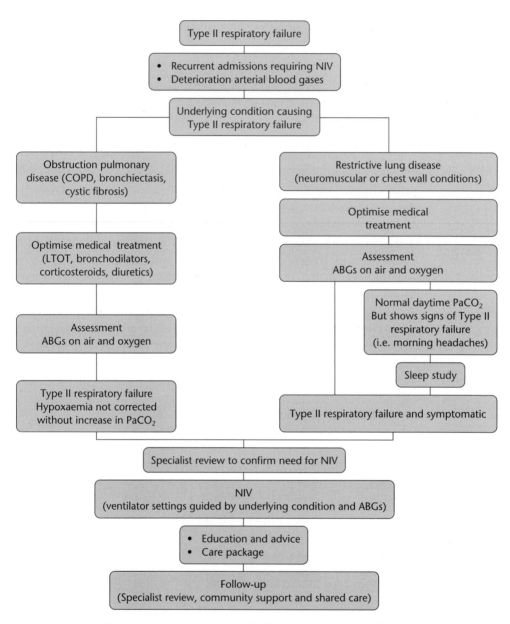

Figure 6.4   Patient selection for home non-invasive ventilation.
COPD, chronic obstructive pulmonary disease; LTOT, long-term oxygen therapy;
ABG, arterial blood gases; NIV, non-invasive ventilation.

Non-invasive Ventilation Healthcare Professional Competency

Healthcare professionals caring for patients on NIV must be trained in its use: this may be a doctor, nurse, physiotherapist or clinical physiologist, provided that they are competent to undertake the procedure, which is an advanced practice. An advanced practice may be defined as an aspect of care which may be undertaken by a qualified healthcare professional who has undergone specific training and assessment, accepts accountability for their actions and feels competent to undertake aspect of care. Before a member of staff may undertake assessment for this practice they must the have completed the following:

1. Agreed with their line manager that it is appropriate to take on this practice as part of their role
2. Attended an NIV workshop or course
3. Gained supervised practice by a member of staff who has been assessed as competent and is undertaking NIV on a regular basis and fulfils the assessment criteria for NIV
4. Assessed as competent in NIV based on criteria below

Activity		Comments
Communication • Able to explain procedure to patient prior to undertaking it • Uses appropriate language when explaining information • Able to develop a plan of care which is clearly documented	☐ ☐ ☐	

Assessment skills
 • Respiratory rate
 • Oxygen saturation
 • Signs of cyanosis
 • Arterial blood gases (states)
    – pre-NIV
    – post-NIV
 • Chest movement
 • Sputum production
	☐
	 ☐
	 ☐
	
	 ☐
	
	 ☐
	 ☐	

Technical skills • Able to set up ventilator • Able to set BPM, IPAP and EPAP settings • Able to choose appropriate mask size • Able to apply nasal/face mask • Able to apply headgear	☐ ☐ ☐ ☐ ☐	

Cognitive
 • Able to interpret arterial blood gases and act on them
 • Able to choose appropriate ventilator settings following assessment
 • Able to troubleshoot complications
    – sores to bridge of nose
    – leaks
    – gastric distension
	☐
	
	 ☐
	
	 ☐	

Patient education • Able to explain to patient rationale for treatment • Able to explain how long the patient needs to use NIV and why	☐ ☐	
I confirm that...has been assessed competent in NIV.		
Assessor's signature:	Date:	

Figure 6.5   Non-invasive ventilation – healthcare professional competency.

covering the essential components of NIV should be completed as this will ensure that staff caring for patients using NIV have the required skills. This will also enable demonstration of clinical governance in relation to the NIV service. This approach is supported by the NHS Knowledge and Skills Framework (Department of Health, 2004). Additional expertise in relation to managing patients at home is required. This includes:

- Assessment of the home environment
- Patient empowerment to improve adherence
- Patient education around recognising signs of deterioration

Patients need to be empowered by healthcare professionals to self-care and become experts in relation to their NIV. To achieve this patients need to be provided with education and support, especially for those going on to use it long-term at home. It is beneficial to have a check list/contract (Figure 6.6) of essential information that needs to be

---

Patient Contract for Using Home NIV

Name...

Address..

....

....

Telephone number...

NHS No...Consultant..........................

I have been shown how to use this equipment	☐
I know how to clean the equipment and the mask	☐
I understand whom to contact should I need help with using NIV	☐
I know the signs and symptoms that might mean that I need to seek assistance from a healthcare professional (i.e. headaches, drowsiness, nasal bridge sore, exacerbation)	☐
I understand that I should come to the emergency department if my condition suddenly deteriorates	☐
I understand that my machine needs servicing once a year and this will be done by the ventilator company	☐
I agree to return the machine when I no longer need it	☐

Signed:..
(Patient)

Countersigned:...
(Healthcare professional)

Figure 6.6 Non-invasive ventilation – patient check list.

covered prior to the patient being sent home with NIV for the first time to reduce clinical risk.

It is also essential that the patient is provided with written information which includes:

- Type of ventilator and serial number
- Mask size and type
- Ventilator settings
- Contact details

A patient information card (Figure 6.7) with this information on it will allow the patient to share this essential information with any healthcare professional involved in their care, particularly if they become acutely ill. Also having contact numbers on a card means it can be left by the telephone in case of emergencies.

Non-Invasive Ventilation Patient Information Card

Name: _____ NHS no: _____

Consultant: _____ Date started NIV: _____

Ventilator type: _____

Serial number: _____

Settings: IPAP: _____ EPAP: _____ BPM: _____ Oxygen: _____

Mask type: _____

In case of breakdown no. nights able to cope without NIV_____

Contact details

Monday to Friday 9 am–5 pm:
In the event of a breakdown or problem with your ventilator, please contact us on:

☎:_____

We will try to assist you over the phone – in the event of an unsolvable problem we can ask the company supplying the machines to deliver a temporary machine within 4 hours.

Out of hours (i.e. 5 pm–9 am Monday to Friday, weekends and Bank Holidays)
If you feel your breathing has or will deteriorate significantly during the above times, you should attend your local emergency department, taking your machine with you. If you feel you do not need to attend as an emergency, but would like to replace a broken machine before the next working day, you can contact:

☎:_____

who will be able to give you a replacement machine. Alternatively, if you feel you can wait until the next working day, please leave a message on our answer phone and we will call you back to sort out the problem:

☎:_____

Servicing
Your machine will be serviced once a year by the supplier, and they will contact you directly regarding visits/appointments to arrange servicing. Their helpline number is ☎:_____(9 am–5 pm Monday to Friday)
please only use this to confirm when your machine will be serviced.

Figure 6.7 Non-invasive ventilation – patient information card.

Audit Record

Patient's name: _____ Hospital number: _____ Date of admission:

Q1   **Sex:**   ☐ Male ☐ Female   **Q2**   **Date of Birth:** ____ /____ /_____

Q3   **Diagnosis:**   ☐ COPD   ☐ Chest wall/neuromuscular
                                     ☐ Obesity/hypoventilation   ☐ Other:
                                       ☐ Cardiogenic pulmonary oedema

           Respiratory failure: ☐ Type 1 (hypoxaemic)   ☐ Type 2 (hypercapnic)

Q4   **Performance status:**   ☐ Normal activity without restriction
                                       ☐ Strenuous activity limited, can do light work
                                       ☐ Limited activity but capable of self care
                                       ☐ Limited activity, limited self care
                                       ☐ Confined to bed/chair, no self care
                                       ☐ No record

Q5   **Focal consolidation on CXR:**   ☐ Yes   ☐ No   ☐ No record

Q6   **Arterial/capillary blood gases:**

	FiO_2 (% or l/min)	PaO_2 (kPa or mmHg)	$PaCO_2$ (kPa or mmHg)	pH (or H^+) (units or nmol/l)
(i) On admission/onset of respiratory failure ☐ No record	_____	_____	_____	_____
(ii) After 1–2 hours of NIV ☐ No record	_____	_____	_____	_____
(iii) After 4–6 hours of NIV ☐ No record	_____	_____	_____	_____
(iv) Pre-discharge ☐ No record	_____	_____	_____	_____

Q7   **Recorded decision on action to be taken if NIV fails:**   ☐ Yes   ☐ No

Q8   **Place where NIV initiated:**   ☐ A&E   ☐ Medical admissions unit
                                  ☐ HDU   ☐ ICU   ☐ Respiratory ward
                                  ☐ General medical ward   ☐ Other:

Q9   **Outcome of NIV:**   ☐ Success/improved
                        ☐ Failure/no benefit
                                 Tracheal intubation   ☐ Yes   ☐ No
                                 Reasons for failure:
                                 ☐ Intolerance of mask   ☐ Excessive secretions
                                 ☐ Nasal bridge erosions   ☐ Other:

Q10   **Complications of NIV:**

Q11   **FEV$_1$:**   ☐ Not done   _____ . _____ litres _____ % predicted

Q12   **Outcome of admissions:**   ☐ Discharged from hospital without NIV
                                  ☐ Discharged from hospital with home NIV
                                  ☐ Died – likely cause of death respiratory
                                  ☐ Died – likely cause of death non-respiratory
                                  ☐ Other:

Q15   **Length of stay:** _____ days   **Q16 Respiratory OPA arranged:**   ☐ Yes ☐ No

Figure 6.8   Audit for acute non-invasive ventilation. Reproduced with permission from the British Thoracic Society Standards of Care Committee (2002) BTS Guideline: Non-invasive ventilation in acute respiratory failure. *Thorax*, **57**, 192–211.

As previously identified, clinical audit is an essential component of service development. In support of this, the British Thoracic Society (2002) NIV Guidelines recommend that all units providing an acute NIV service should record clinical outcomes of patients using NIV. This will allow care standards to be monitored within the organisation. This can be used as part of national audits (Figure 6.8), allowing benchmarking of care to ensure best practice is achieved equitably.

The audit for patients using NIV long-term at home needs to be more focused on the patient's experience, because their ability to cope independently with the NIV will improve adherence with the treatment. Outcomes covering the key clinical issues that are measurable by either asking, observing or checking can be developed and used as the audit criteria for evaluating the quality of the home NIV service (Figure 6.9).

Target group	Method	Audit criteria	Yes/No
Patient/carer	Ask	Has the patient been provided with training and can they state the purpose of the treatment?	
Patient/carer	Ask/observe	Does the patient have written information about their NIV?	
Patient/carer	Ask/observe	Is the patient comfortable during the procedure and had sensations related to NIV explained?	
Patient/carer	Ask/observe	Can patient and/or carer independently put on NIV mask and switch on machine?	
Patient/carer	Ask/observe	Does the patient know the contact numbers and whom to contact for: • Clinical advice • Mechanical breakdown	
Staff	Records	Is patient's response to therapy recorded?	
Staff	Check	Is the equipment stored and kept clean by patient and annual servicing carried out?	
Patient	Ask	Can patient state how to recognise signs of deterioration? • Headache • Drowsiness • Flushing • Exacerbation	
Patient	Ask/observe	Has patient any complications of NIV? • Nasal bridge sore • Gastric distension • Conjunctivitis • Rhinitis	

Figure 6.9 Audit for home non-invasive ventilation and continuous positive airway pressure (CPAP).

Home oxygen

Home oxygen therapy involves the provision of either long-term oxygen therapy (LTOT), ambulatory oxygen, and, for a small number of patients, short-burst oxygen therapy (SBOT) outside the hospital setting, which could be the patient's home, relative/friends home, residential care home or holiday destinations. To ensure that appropriate patients receive home oxygen, clear clinical decision making, based on guidelines and evidence, is necessary.

Clinical decision making, protocols and standards of care

The key consideration of the clinical decision-making process is the assessment, safety, patient education and follow-up. The aim of an oxygen therapy service is to ensure that all patients who meet the criteria for home oxygen therapy are provided with the most appropriate modality (LTOT, SBOT, ambulatory), at the correct flow rate and duration, in a timely and safe way. To meet the patient's needs, the home oxygen service requires the following components:

- Referral process
- Assessment
- Liaison with delivery service/oxygen company
- Patient education including safety with oxygen
- Follow-up service including a register of patients on home oxygen
- Monitoring of service and clinical audit

When setting up a home oxygen service, existing patients on home oxygen within the local area should be identified. This will allow an analysis of the numbers of patients requiring the service, which will inform the level of resource needed. Also the breakdown between LTOT, ambulatory and SBOT can be established, which will allow anomalies in oxygen prescribing to be identified, for example, high level of SBOT usually indicates that patients have not been formally assessed. This will allow priorities to be identified and an action plan developed. The plan should include:

- Resources (staff and equipment).
- Referral criteria for assessment including referral form.
- Communication of assessment results, decisions and actions.

Table 6.1 Components of home oxygen service.

What	Who	Where	How
Screening to identify patients requiring referral for oxygen assessment ($SpO_2 < 92\%$)	Primary care health professional (e.g. GP, practice nurse, district nurse, community matron)	Primary care: • GP new patient screening • Home visits by community nurses • Annual review	Pulse oximeter
Assessment for long-term oxygen therapy (LTOT) ($SpO_2 < 92\%$)	Specialist respiratory healthcare professional	Secondary care or community hospital	• Blood gas machine that is maintained for quality • Expertise to interpret blood gases • Oxygen concentrator
Assessment for ambulatory oxygen for mobile patients on LTOT or those who have oxygen desaturation on exercise	Specialist respiratory healthcare professional	Secondary care or community hospital	• Expertise to perform 6-minute or shuttle walk test • Room to undertake walk test • Ambulatory oxygen cylinders • Pulse oximeter • Stop watch
Follow-up appointment in the home within 4 weeks	Specialist respiratory or primary care health professional	Patient's home	• Appointment • Pulse oximeter
Follow-up appointment at 3 months	Specialist respiratory or primary care health professional	Patient's home or at outpatient clinic	• Appointment • Pulse oximeter
Continuing patient follow-up in the home	Primary care health professional	Patient's home	• Appointment • Pulse oximeter
• Annual review • Spirometry • Arterial blood gases • Review of medication • Assessment of impact of living with oxygen	Specialist respiratory healthcare professional	Secondary care or community hospital	• Blood gas machine that is maintained for quality • Spirometer • Expertise in respiratory disease management

- Patient information and education on home oxygen individually tailored to the individual.
- Communication of follow-up and any changes made to oxygen therapy.

Breaking down the various components of the home oxygen service allows the facilities, staffing and equipment to be identified (Table 6.1). This can be used to form the foundation of the business case to support the development of the home oxygen service.

Once resources have been agreed as identified in Table 6.1 there is a need to inform healthcare professionals about the service which can be achieved through educational events, direct mail, newsletter articles and the use of the intranet. The main messages that need to be communicated are:

- The reason for the service.
- Why it is important to assess patients with a SaO_2 less than 92%.
- The benefits of following up patients on home oxygen.
- Criteria for referral.
- How to refer to assessment and follow-up service.

To facilitate this, a flow diagram (Figure 6.10), outlining the process from screening to follow-up, and a referral form (Figure 6.11), which includes the referral criteria, are required so that appropriate referrals are received and that there is a clear pathway that can be audited against.

Home oxygen is only one aspect of the care required to treat underlying respiratory disease, therefore it is important that healthcare professional assessing and managing patients on home oxygen use this opportunity to review the underlying condition as well. To ensure that patients requiring home oxygen receive quality care it is essential that healthcare professionals have knowledge and skills in screening, assessing, managing and monitoring patients when oxygen is indicated in accordance with evidence-based guidelines. To achieve this, healthcare professionals should have access to educational programmes and complete a competency assessment (Figure 6.12), covering the essential components of oxygen therapy ensuring that staff caring for patients on home oxygen have the required skills.

Patients initiated on oxygen therapy often find this a difficult time as they are often coming to come to terms with acceptance of deteriorating health and also coping with the addition of oxygen in their daily life. It is therefore necessary to provide patients with information about

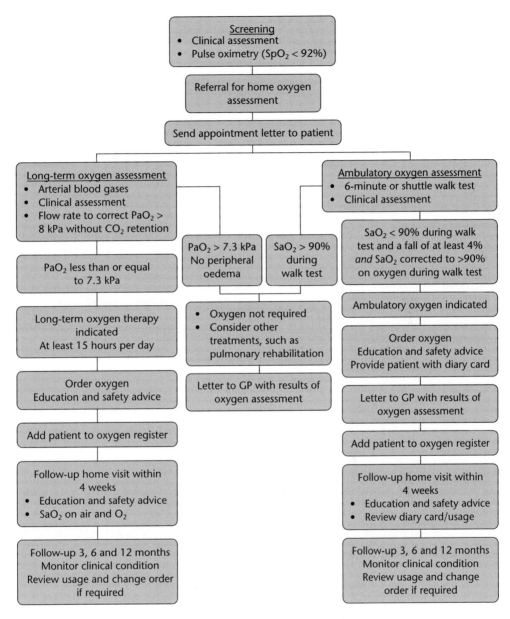

Figure 6.10 Home oxygen – patient selection.

Referral for Home Oxygen Assessment	
Type of oxygen referral being requested: **Long-term oxygen therapy** ☐ (tick if required) **Ambulatory oxygen referral** ☐ (tick if required)	Send referral form to:
Patient name: NHS number: Date of birth: Patient address: Phone number:	GP: Address: Tel no:
Respiratory diagnosis: _____ Co-morbidities: Angina Yes/No CHD Yes/No Recent MI Yes/No Falls Yes/No Other:	SaO$_2$ _____% (if available) Current mobility: Distance: _____ Use of aids: _____ Has patient attended pulmonary rehabilitation Yes/No
Referred by: _____ Date: _____	
Contact details/Surgery stamp	

Long-term oxygen referral criteria	**Ambulatory oxygen referral criteria**
• SaO$_2$ less than 92% on air at rest • 5 weeks post exacerbation	• On long-term oxygen therapy • Goes out of home and willing to use oxygen outside OR • Not on long-term oxygen therapy but breathless on exercise

Figure 6.11   Home oxygen – referral form.

their home oxygen therapy. Common questions asked by patients are outlined in Box 6.1.

The audit for patients using oxygen therapy at home needs to focus on the patient's experience, because their ability to cope independently with the oxygen will improve adherence with the treatment. Outcomes covering the key clinical issues that are measurable by either asking,

---

Home Oxygen Healthcare Professional Competency Assessment

Healthcare professionals caring for patients on home oxygen therapy must be trained in its use. Registered practitioners must be competent to assess, deliver and monitor patients requiring LTOT, ambulatory and SBOT prior to being able to prescribe/order home oxygen. Healthcare professionals should be assessed as competent in home oxygen therapy based on the criteria below.

Activity		Comments
Communication • Able to explain criteria for referring patients for an oxygen assessment to healthcare professionals • Able to explain reasons for LTOT and ambulatory oxygen assessment and what they involve • Able to develop a plan of care which is clearly documented • Able to complete oxygen order form effectively communicate with oxygen company	☐ ☐ ☐ ☐	
Assessment skills • Able to state when to carry out an oxygen assessment • Able to assess for risk factors prior to performing ambulatory oxygen assessment • Able to perform pulse oximetry • Able to state when and why pulse oximetry should be performed and its limitations • Able to state when and why arterial/arterialised blood gases need to be performed	☐ ☐ ☐ ☐ ☐	
Technical skills • Able to perform LTOT assessment • Able to undertake 6-minute walk test and/or shuttle walk test • Able to perform and/or order arterial/arterialised blood gases	☐ ☐ ☐	
Cognitive • Able to interpret arterial/arterialised blood gases and act on them • Able to interpret walk test results • Able to choose appropriate modality of oxygen therapy (LTOT, SBOT, ambulatory) • Able to determine flow rate and hours of usage • Uses research and clinical guidelines to inform practice	☐ ☐ ☐ ☐ ☐	
Patient education • Able to explain to patient rationale for treatment • Able to explain how long the patient needs to use the oxygen • Able to explain safety aspects when using oxygen therapy	☐ ☐ ☐	
I confirm that...has been assessed competent in home oxygen therapy. Assessor's signature: Date:		

Figure 6.12 Home oxygen – competency. LTOT, long-term oxygen therapy; SBOT, short-burst oxygen therapy.

Box 6.1 Oxygen in the home – what you need to know. Patient education – questions and answers.

Oxygen is a drug that can only be prescribed by a qualified healthcare professional. It can be provided by cylinders or by an oxygen concentrator machine. If you have been prescribed oxygen for use in the home you need to know the following.

Why do I need oxygen treatment?

Oxygen is essential for life and healthy lungs can extract enough oxygen from the air for normal body requirements. In lung disease, this process is impaired and can result in low blood oxygen levels. Oxygen is prescribed to correct a low oxygen level in the blood and is given to patients who have various lung diseases.

How much oxygen will I need?

To decide how much oxygen (litres per minute) and for how long (hours per day) you need to be assessed. This will include having blood taken from an artery while breathing air and oxygen.

Can I overdose on oxygen?

It is very important that you only use your prescribed dose of oxygen. More oxygen is not necessarily better for you, in fact it may be dangerous and cause you harm. Too much oxygen can cause the carbon dioxide level in your blood to rise. This can cause excessive sleepiness, headaches, confusion and disorientation.

Is oxygen safe?

Provided that you **do not smoke** while on oxygen and that you use the oxygen at the prescribe level then it is safe. It is important that you **do not smoke** as this may cause a fire.

How is oxygen provided in the home?

The most convenient way of providing oxygen in the home is via an oxygen concentrator as it runs off the electricity supply therefore does not run out. Sometimes cylinders are supplied if oxygen is only used intermittently, although this is only occasionally indicated. For patients who require oxygen to get out of the home, small portable cylinders can be provided. Once you have been assessed for home oxygen it will be ordered and then delivered to your home by the oxygen supplier.

What is an oxygen concentrator?

This is an electrically operated machine that draws in room air and converts it into oxygen by removing the nitrogen and other gases.

Can I have an oxygen concentrator?

Specific assessment must be performed and results must comply with guidelines before the specialist can advise on prescription. The oxygen concentrator is prescribed and ordered by the specialist doctor or nurse to a supplier who will arrange for its delivery and installation in your home.

Is the oxygen treatment different from a concentrator?

This prescription requires a minimum of 15 hours oxygen a day and is given to improve the function of the heart, prolong life and correct low oxygen levels in the blood. It is not given primarily to relieve breathlessness. Delivery via nasal prongs makes this treatment more acceptable. Oxygen from a concentrator may feel different to cylinder because it is not pressurised but it is the same concentration of oxygen.

What is ambulatory oxygen?

This is the use of small portable oxygen cylinders while walking or exercising.

Can I have a portable oxygen cylinder?

Specific assessment must be performed involving a walking test to determine if you drop your oxygen levels when mobile and what flow rate (litres/minute) is required. If you require ambulatory oxygen the portable cylinders will be prescribed and ordered by the specialist doctor or nurse to a supplier who will arrange for its delivery.

How do I get another portable cylinder of oxygen?

The supplier will continue to deliver oxygen to your home as prescribed by your doctor or nurse. You will be given a telephone number by the supplier when you get your first delivery and all you do is phone the supplier when you need a replacement and they will arrange delivery.

Do I need regular check ups if I use oxygen?

Guidelines produced by respiratory specialists recommend that anyone who uses oxygen at home should be visited at home within a few weeks of starting oxygen and then reviewed at least 6 monthly thereafter.

Target group	Method	Audit criteria	Yes/No
Staff	Ask/check	Is the patient on the oxygen register?	
Staff	Records/check	Is there a documented home oxygen assessment?	
Patient/carer	Ask/observe	Does the patient have written information about how to use their home oxygen?	
Patient/carer	Ask	Does patient know flow rate and hours per day that oxygen should be used?	
Patient/carer	Ask	Does patient know risk of smoking while on oxygen?	
Patient/carer	Ask/records	Was the patient visited at home within 4 weeks of commencing home oxygen?	
Patient/carer	Ask/observe	Can patient and/or carer independently use oxygen?	
Patient/carer	Ask/observe	Does the patient know the contact numbers and whom to contact for: • Clinical advice • Mechanical breakdown	
Staff	Records	Is patient's response to therapy recorded?	
Patient/carer	Check	Is the equipment positioned appropriately in the home?	
Patient	Ask	Can patient state how to recognise signs of acute exacerbation?	

Figure 6.13 Home oxygen – audit criteria.

observing or checking can be developed and used as the audit criteria for evaluating the quality of the home oxygen service (Figure 6.13). In addition the database that forms the register of patients on home oxygen within a region can be used to benchmark its modality break-down and usage against population data and also national trends.

Home CPAP for sleep apnoea

The use of home CPAP in the context of service delivery is where the patient has CPAP at home overnight to treat obstructive sleep apnoea/hypopnoea syndrome. It should only be given following a full assessment, including sleep studies, to evaluate response to CPAP in accordance with guidelines (Scottish Intercollegiate Guidelines Network (SIGN),

2003; NICE, 2008). In addition, an assessment must be made of the patient's ability to manage the machine independently. The patient needs to be educated and advised about its safe use, and many patients will also need to lose weight as obesity is one of the most common reasons for obstructive sleep apnoea/hypopnoea syndrome. Therefore behaviour modification to assist the patient with adherence may be required and the healthcare professional will need to support the patient particularly in the early stages of commencing CPAP. Table 6.2 outlines the various components of the sleep service from diagnosis to follow-up.

Clinical decision making, protocols and standards of care

The key consideration of the clinical decision making when providing a home CPAP service is assessment, provision and maintenance of equipment and patient safety. The aim of a home CPAP service is to ensure that all patients who meet the criteria for CPAP are provided with well-maintained equipment set at the correct pressure to prevent the upper airway obstructing during sleep. To meet the patient's needs the home CPAP service requires the following components:

- Assessment (differential diagnosis confirmed by sleep studies)
- Patient information and education
- Patient and public safety (driving and alcohol use)
- Follow-up to review patient's need to continue as some patients when they lose weight may no longer obstruct their airway
- Monitoring of service and clinical audit

Figure 6.14 shows the patient selection and clinical pathway for CPAP.

Staff competency and education

Patients requiring home CPAP are usually not as ill as those requiring NIV, however, for the patient and their family it can be difficult to adjust to using the CPAP machine overnight. If patients are not provided with sufficient information and education about the use of CPAP, they may not adhere to the treatment. This is supported by Lin et al. (2007), who demonstrated in their study that non-compliance with CPAP is 37%. On the other hand, it has been found that where additional support has

Table 6.2 Components of home CPAP service.

What	Who	Where	How
Screening to identify patients requiring referral for assessment and sleep study	• Primary care health professional (e.g. GP) • Occupational health	Primary care: • GP new patient screening • Patient symptomatic	• Clinical assessment • Epworth score >10 • Body mass index
Assessment for obstructive sleep apnoea/hypopnoea syndrome	Specialist respiratory/sleep health professional	Secondary or community care	• Sleep study • Expertise to interpret sleep study
Provision of CPAP equipment	Specialist respiratory/sleep healthcare professional	Secondary or community care	• Expertise to set up CPAP • Education and advice
Follow-up appointment after 3 months	Specialist respiratory/sleep or primary care health professional	Secondary or community care	• Appointment
• Annual review • Spirometry • Arterial blood gases • Review of medication • Assessment of impact of living with CPAP • Nutritional advice	Specialist respiratory/sleep health professional	Secondary or community care	• Blood gas machine that is maintained for quality • Spirometer • Expertise in respiratory/sleep disease management

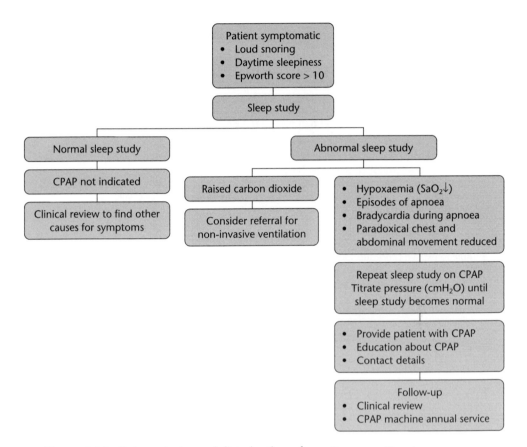

Figure 6.14 Patient selection and clinical pathway for continuous positive airway pressure.

been given, compliance with CPAP can be achieved in 95% of patients (Chervin et al., 1997). It is therefore essential that the staff involved in the CPAP service have the skills and are competent in its use. Figure 6.15 provides a competency assessment that could be used in conjunction with an education programme.

Patients also require education and information about the use of CPAP; besides verbal instructions, the patient should also be provided with written information. Box 6.2 is an example of a question and answer approach to providing information.

Audit of the CPAP service will be necessary to ensure that the quality of the service is monitored and any aspects identified as requiring attention are addressed through an action plan. The audit criteria for CPAP and NIV are similar as essentially the same principles of care apply (see Figure 6.9).

CPAP Healthcare Professional Competency Assessment

Healthcare professionals caring for patients requiring CPAP must be trained in its use: this may be a doctor, nurse, physiotherapist or clinical physiologist provided that they are competent to undertake the procedure, which is an advanced practice. An advanced practice may be defined as an aspect of care which may be undertaken by a qualified healthcare professional who has undergone specific training and assessment, accepts accountability for their actions and feels competent to undertake the aspect of care. Before a member of staff may undertake assessment for this practice they must have completed the following:

1. Agreed with their line manager that it is appropriate to take on this practice as part of their role
2. Attended a CPAP workshop or course
3. Gained supervised practice by a member of staff who has been assessed as competent and is undertaking CPAP on a regular basis and fulfils the assessment criteria for CPAP
4. Assessed as competent in CPAP based on criteria below

Activity		Comments
Communication • Able to explain procedures to patient prior to undertaking it • Uses appropriate language when explaining information • Able to develop a plan of care which is clearly documented	☐ ☐ ☐	
Assessment skills • Respiratory rate • Oxygen saturation • Signs of cyanosis • Arterial blood gases • Chest movement	☐ ☐ ☐ ☐ ☐	
Technical skills • Able to set up CPAP machine • Able to set CPAP pressure • Able to choose appropriate mask size • Able to apply nasal/face mask • Able to apply headgear	☐ ☐ ☐ ☐ ☐	

Cognitive
• Able to interpret sleep study
• Able to choose appropriate CPAP pressure (mmH$_2$O) following assessment
• Able to troubleshoot complications
  – sores to bridge of nose
  – leaks
  – gastric distension
	☐
	☐
	
	☐	

Patient education • Able to explain to patient rationale for treatment • Able to explain how long the patient needs to use CPAP and why	☐ ☐	
I confirm that...has been assessed competent in CPAP.		
Assessor's signature:	Date:	

Figure 6.15 Continuous positive airway pressure – competency assessment.

Box 6.2 Continuous positive airway pressure – questions and answers. Management of obstructive sleep apnoea/hypopnoea syndrome in adults.

Information for discussion with patients and carers.

The following sample information sheet can be used in discussion with patients to highlight issues of particular importance. It is intended as a guide only and should not be used to plan treatment or to replace the important consultations that should be held between patients and healthcare professionals.

What is sleep apnoea/hypopnoea syndrome?

People who suffer from obstructive sleep apnoea/hypopnoea syndrome (OSAHS) breathe shallowly or stop breathing for short periods while sleeping. This can happen many times during the night. It results in poor sleep leading to excessive sleepiness during the day. Because these events occur during sleep, a person suffering from OSAHS is often the last one to know what is happening.

In deep sleep, the muscles of the throat relax. Normally this doesn't cause any problems with breathing. In OSAHS, complete relaxation of the throat muscles causes blockage of the upper airway at the back of the tongue. Normal breathing then slows or stops completely. Such an episode is called an apnoea. During an apnoea, people with OSAHS make constant efforts to breathe against their blocked airway until the blood oxygen level begins to fall. The brain then needs to arouse the person from deep relaxed sleep so that the muscle tone returns, the upper airway then opens and breathing begins again. Unfortunately, when a person with OSAHS falls back into deep sleep, the muscles relax once more and the cycle repeats itself again and again overnight.

In OSAHS, the apnoeas can last for several seconds and in severe cases the cycle of apnoeas and broken sleep is repeated hundreds of times per night. Most sufferers are unaware of their disrupted sleep but awaken unrefreshed, feeling sleepy and in need of further refreshing sleep.

Who gets OSAHS?

Whilst OSAHS is more common in overweight middle-aged males who snore, it can also affect females, although female hormones and a difference in throat structures may protect women until the menopause. Narrowing of the back of the throat and the upper airway can also contribute to the risk of getting OSAHS, even in people who are not overweight or middle-aged. In such people a small jaw, enlarged tongue, big tonsils and big soft palate help to block the upper airway

Box 6.2 Continued

in deep sleep, making OSAHS more likely to occur. Several of these problems can be present in any person at the same time.

The use of alcohol, sleeping tablets and tranquillisers prior to sleep relaxes the upper airway muscles and make OSAHS worse. Alcohol can also reduce the brain's response to an apnoea which in turn leads to longer and more severe apnoeas in people who would otherwise have only mild OSAHS and who would otherwise only snore.

What are the symptoms of OSAHS?

Most people with OSAHS snore loudly and breathing during sleep may be laboured and noisy. Sleeping partners may report multiple apnoeas which often end in deep gasping and loud snorting. Sufferers may report waking for short periods after struggling for breath. Symptoms are often worse when lying on the back in deepest sleep.

Although a person with OSAHS may not be aware of the many arousals from deep sleep, they suffer from poor quality sleep in spite of long periods of time spent in bed. Such people wake feeling that they haven't had a full refreshing night's sleep. They report difficulty maintaining concentration during the day, have a poor memory, and suffer from excessive daytime sleepiness.

At first an OSAHS sufferer may be sleepy only when seated and relaxed, e.g. watching TV, but eventually sleepiness becomes so severe that car accidents and accidents in the workplace occur. Other symptoms of OSAHS include morning headache, nocturia, depression, short temper, grumpiness, personality change, and impotence in males, leading to loss of interest in sex.

What are the consequences of untreated OSAHS?

The most serious potential consequences of untreated OSAHS are road traffic accidents and accidents at work because of sleepiness. Untreated OSAHS is associated with a sixfold increase in risk of such accidents. Patients may also experience difficulties with concentration due to tiredness, increased irritability and depression. There is evidence that patients with OSAHS have an increased risk of high blood pressure and may have a slightly increased risk of angina, heart attacks and strokes. Because OSAHS significantly increases the risk of road traffic accidents patients must not drive if experiencing excessive daytime sleepiness. Patients must inform the DVLA in Swansea following a diagnosis of the condition. In most cases, the DVLA are happy to allow car drivers to continue driving once they are established on a successful therapy.

How is OSAHS assessed?

When a person is suspected to have OSAHS, their doctor will ask questions about waking and sleeping habits and will make a physical examination. Reports from the sleeping partner or household member about any apnoeas are extremely helpful.

Referral to a sleep disorders centre for an overnight sleep study will probably be required to confirm the diagnosis of OSAHS and to allow its severity to be measured.

During a sleep study, sleep quality and breathing are measured overnight by a computer while the person sleeps. Procedures in different hospitals vary but small coin-sized electrodes may be taped to special points on the scalp, face, chest and legs. Chest and stomach wall movements are also measured and a special sensor placed on the upper lip measures airflow. The oxygen level in the blood is assessed by a device placed on the finger or the earlobe. None of these procedures are uncomfortable or painful.

How is OSAHS treated?

The simplest treatment is to lose weight. This is best done by cutting down on all foods, especially fatty foods, sweet things and alcohol. Alcohol within six hours of bedtime should be avoided as it contributes to OSAHS symptoms. If these measures are not enough, the best form of treatment is continuous positive airway pressure (CPAP) therapy in which a gentle flow of air is applied through the nose at night keeping the pressure in the throat above atmospheric pressure and stopping the throat narrowing to prevent breathing pauses and snoring.

Other forms of treatment include gumshield-like devices (mandibular repositioning devices) which attempt to keep the airway clear by moving the jaw forward. Surgery to remove excess tissue from the throat is another option, but it is not recommended. Both of these alternatives are less effective than CPAP and not appropriate for all patients.

Reproduced with permission from the Scottish Intercollegiate Guidelines Network: Management of Obstructive of Sleep Apnoea/Hypopnoea Syndrome in Adults (June 2003).

Service development

Respiratory support services, whether new or being developed further in line with changing clinical and patients needs, require to be based on a business case as this will allow services to be considered by commissioners. An important aspect of the business case is the costing of the service so that resources are identified to provide a quality service. Figures 6.16 is a template for a service improvement plan that allows the service development to be planned using objectives and outcomes. This approach allows the development to be project managed and can be then used to form the basis of the business case. Figure 6.17 is a template of a business case that identifies the type of information that needs to be included.

Objectives	Outcomes	Actions	Responsibility	Timescale	Progress
Project Lead:		Project Sponsor:			
Objective 1					
Objective 2					
Objective 3					
Objective 4					
Objective 5					

Figure 6.16   Service improvement plan.

Business Case
PROJECT TITLE:
Background and justification for change:
Link to Strategic Fit:
Aims and description of Proposal:
Initial Risks:
Expected Outcomes:
Benefits of this Project:
Existing Activity Levels and Costs:
The Project will increase activity and the financial implications are:
Estimates of Full Cost of Project:
Timescales:
Name of person completing Business Case:
Outcome of Business Case:
Decision to be made at:
Date:

Figure 6.17 Business case template.

References

British Thoracic Society Standards of Care Committee (2002) BTS Guideline: Non-invasive ventilation in acute respiratory failure. *Thorax*, **57**, 192–211.

Chervin, R.D., Theut, S., Bassetti, C. & Aldrich, M.S. (1997) Compliance with nasal CPAP can be improved with simple interventions. *Sleep*, **20**, 284–289.

Department of Health (2000) *Comprehensive Critical Care: A Review of Adult Critical Care Service*. The Stationery Office, London.

Department of Health (2001) *The Expert Patient: A New Approach to Chronic Disease Management for the 21st Century*. The Stationery Office, London.

Department of Health (2004) *The NHS Knowledge and Skills Framework (NHS KSF) and the Development Review Process*. The Stationery Office, London.

Department of Health (2006) *Gold Standard Framework: a Programme for Community Palliative Care*. The Stationery Office, London.

Kennedy, I. (2001) *The Report of the Public Inquiry into Children's Heart Surgery at the Bristol Royal Infirmary 1984–1995. Learning From Bristol*. The Stationery Office, London.

Lin, H-S., Prasad, A.S., Pan, C-J.G. & Rowley, J.A. (2007) Factors associated with noncompliance to treatment with positive airway pressure. *Archives of Otolaryngology, Head and Neck Surgery*, **133**, 69–72.

Liverpool Care Pathway for the Dying Patient (LCP) (2004) Available at: http://www.mcpcil.org.uk/liverpool_care_pathway (accessed 9 May 2008).

Meecham-Jones, D.J., Paul, E.A., Jones, P.W. & Wedzicha, J.A. (1995) Nasal pressure support ventilation plus oxygen compared with oxygen therapy alone in hypercapnic COPD. *American Journal of Respiratory and Critical Care Medicine*, **152**, 538–544.

National Institute for Health and Clinical Excellence (NICE) (2008) Continuous positive airway pressure for the treatment of obstructive sleep apnoea/hypopnoea syndrome. Technical appraisal 139. NICE, London. Available at: www.nice.org.uk/ta139 (accessed 17 May 2008).

National Institute of Clinical Excellence (2002) *Principles of Best Practice in Clinical Audit*. NICE, London.

Plant, P.K., Owen, J.L. & Elliott, M.W. (2000) Early use of non-invasive ventilation for acute exacerbations of chronic obstructive pulmonary disease on general respiratory wards: a multicentre randomised controlled trial. *Lancet*, **355**, 1931–1935.

Royal College of Nursing (2003) *Clinical Governance: an RCN Resource Guide*. Royal College of Nursing, London.

Scally, G. & Donaldson, L.J. (1998) Clinical governance and the drive for quality improvement in the new NHS in England. *British Medical Journal*, **317**, 61–65.

Scottish Intercollegiate Guidelines Network (2003) Management of obstructive sleep apnoea/hypopnoea syndrome in adults. A national clinical guideline. SIGN, Edinburgh.

Chapter 7

ETHICS

This chapter considers the ethical and legal aspects of decision making in relation to non-invasive respiratory support techniques in the clinical setting. The main issues covered include:

- Principle-based approach to ethical decision making
- End-of-life decisions including withdrawal of treatment, resuscitation status and advance directives
- Ethical clinical decision making
- Legal cases to support decision making

Principle-based approach to ethical decision making

The use of a principle-based approach as described by Beauchamp & Childress (2001) considers ethical problems in terms of respect for:

- **Autonomy**: the obligation to respect the decision-making abilities of autonomous people.
- **Beneficence**: the obligation to provide benefits and balance against risk.
- **Non-maleficence**: the obligation to avoid causing harm.
- **Justice**: the obligation to distribute benefits and risks fairly.

The principle-based approach allows for the consideration of moral issues from a number of perspectives and provides a strategy for ethical decision making (Edwards, 1996). This is especially relevant in end-of-life decisions which are fraught with ethical and emotional problems. The principles that are relevant to our dilemma of withdrawal of treatment are respect for autonomy, beneficence and non-maleficence, and each need to be considered in relation to the deontological and utilitarian approaches (Table 7.1).

Table 7.1 Deontological and utilitarian approaches.

Theory	Approach	Strengths
Deontology	Deontology takes as its primary premise that there are certain indisputable, fixed duties – a premise reflected in the roots of the world's religions. Kant proposed that humanity should be treated never as simply a means, but always as an end. He considered that the 'mind' should be free to make moral decisions and that autonomy in pursuit of moral duty was central to moral thought. The consideration of consequences of actions was deemed to be a threat to autonomy (Edwards, 1996)	Strengths of the Kantian theory are that it recognises the importance of individuals as equals and advocates a right that is recognised by the majority as being a right (Singleton & McLaren, 1995). Criticisms of this theory have centred on its absolutism. Kant was unequivocal in that the supreme moral law applied categorically and without exception (Gillon, 1985). In addition, the inflexibility of Kant's philosophy makes it difficult to apply to the dynamic healthcare environment where compromise may be essential for 'good' patient care and where consequences of actions must be taken into account (Seedhouse, 1998)
Utilitarianism	Utilitarianism is described as 'the greatest happiness of the greatest number' (Bentham, 1789; Mill 1861, cited in Ryan, 1987) **Act-utilitarianism** States that a person must assess how their actions could produce the best balance of good over evil in each new situation without recourse to rules or principles, although they must take into account the possible effect on others (Seedhouse, 1998) **Rule-utilitarianism** Rule-utilitarians use an indirect approach that employs rules which have a utilitarian justification to produce a good outcome (Singleton & McLaren, 1995)	The strengths of utilitarianism lie in the fact that it does not rely on moral intuitions, as Kantian deontology does, because of its belief that happiness is good and suffering is evil and that it offers a consistent process for making moral decisions (Gillon, 1985). Also, as a principle based on the greatest good for all, it has a positive resonance with many working in a public health system (Seedhouse, 1998)

Autonomous choice is a fundamental obligation of healthcare workers in ensuring that patients have the right to choose and accept or refuse information or treatment. The philosophies of both Kant and Mill support the principle of respect for autonomy but in different ways (Beauchamp & Childress, 2001). Kant's moral imperative is to respect autonomy of will, while Mill is concerned with autonomy of thought and action and requires that an individual's autonomous expression is not interfered with and is actively strengthened, as long as it does not interfere with the expression of freedom of others. Both agree with respect for autonomy and much of healthcare is about the restoration of autonomy (Edwards, 1996). However, as Brooks (1997) points out, there are many situations, such as the withdrawal of treatment, where autonomy may not be exercised because of physical or mental incapacity. One way of overcoming this dilemma is by patients making their wishes known through an advance directive, before they become incapacitated.

Utilitarianism values respect the autonomy of the individual only to the extent that it will increase utility and Mill (1861, cited in Ryan, 1987) excluded those who were unable to look after themselves – which may include terminally ill patients on non-invasive ventilation (Singleton & McLaren, 1995). Kant's principle of respect for autonomy requires a level of rationality so those without it will be excluded from the range of the principle (Gillon, 1985). However, Fraser & Walters (2000) defend the right of any patient to participate in end-of-life decisions, an opinion mirrored by Gillon (2003), who stated that respect for autonomy was 'first among equals' of the four ethical principles of:

- Autonomy
- Beneficence
- Non-maleficence
- Justice

Autonomy

The issue of the quality of a patient's understanding and consent in relation to autonomous choice has been raised by many ethicists. Dare (1998) views the availability of sufficient information as vital in order to protect an individual's autonomous choice. Therefore, competence in decision making by patients is closely related to autonomous decision making and a judgement of competence may be required to determine whether a patient's decision should be overridden. Patients could be judged to be competent if they can understand information, make judgements about it in the light of their values, intend a specific outcome and can communicate their wishes (Beauchamp & Childress, 2001).

Patients using non-invasive ventilation may be cognitively impaired by drugs or hypoxaemia. Cognitive impairment is a resultant consequence of hypoxaemia and has been demonstrated by Liesker et al. (2004) as having a significant impact on these patients in relation to cognition. In addition, patients may not be in a position to communicate effectively because of the continuous use of a nasal or face mask and may therefore not be in a position to decide autonomously whether they should continue with treatment or not. As Beauchamp and Childress (2001) point out, assessment of competence is fraught with difficulty. However, the utilitarian view that autonomy is only valued if the best outcome can be achieved, would support the giving of incomplete information to achieve this end (Singleton & McLaren, 1995).

If it is not possible to apply the principle of respect for autonomy as a result of incompetence of a patient, a paternalistic intervention could be supported, on the grounds of beneficence, such as treating the patient in their best interests (Dare, 1998). In circumstances where a patient is unable to communicate his or her wishes and their former requests are unknown, surrogate decision makers, which may include healthcare workers and family members, must consider what is in the patient's best interests – either based on what the patient would have decided if they were competent or on the value the patient would place on their own life in the given situation (Lazar et al., 1996; Dare, 1998). The benefits and harms of treatments must be weighed against each other to determine their overall effectiveness (Beauchamp & Childress, 2001) and an assessment of the quality of life that a patient may expect, following treatment, may also play an important and challenging part in decision making (Dare, 1998).

Beneficence and non-maleficence

Some view beneficence and non-maleficence as poles of the same continuum, but the difficulty here is that there is a universal duty not to harm, whereas there is latitude in whom we help (Beauchamp & Childress, 2001). Kant describes the duty of non-maleficence as a 'perfect duty' while beneficence is an 'imperfect duty' (Kant, cited in Singleton & McLaren, 1995, p. 41). Non-maleficence encompasses the doctrine of double effect, which is supported by Kantian philosophy. It is not considered maleficent to withdraw treatments such as non-invasive ventilation, when to continue would cause further pain, distress or burden, or when the likelihood of benefit or survival is poor (Lloyd, 1989). This raises the issue of how and by whom futility of medical interventions is assessed (Dare, 1998) and the issue of ordinary and extra-ordinary treatments for which there have been no absolute definitions (Beauchamp & Childress, 2001). The use of non-invasive ventilation could be considered to be an extra-ordinary measure because it provides ventilatory support although it is not a complex treatment to apply.

Utilitarians would argue that once the decision is made that death is the best outcome, then the patient should be killed rather than letting the patient die, as that would be less painful for the patient, family and the healthcare workers involved (Singleton & McLaren, 1995). However, this point of view does not take into account the legal implications, as euthanasia remains illegal in many countries.

End-of-life decisions

End-of-life decision making is complex, although if ethical principles are applied this will allow clarity of the process. The principles that need to be considered are:

- Sanctity of life
- Slippery slope argument
- Doctrine of double effect
- Distinction between acts and omissions

Sanctity of life

When considering end-of-life issues the principle of sanctity of life requires exploration because of the range of perspectives which different philosophical viewpoints offer and because of its importance to the English legal system (Skene & Parker, 2002). The Western traditional view of the sanctity of life is a blend of Christian, Jewish and Greek religious influences (Rachels, 1986) and over the ages there have been differing points of view (Table 7.2). Utilitarians were the first to provide a principled defence of euthanasia (Rachels, 1986). Bentham (cited in Ryan, 1987) supported the view that if misery was decreased by providing a quick and painless death for those dying in agony then that was

Table 7.2 Changing beliefs in sanctity to life.

Period	Beliefs
Early Christians	Against the killing of human beings in any circumstance, including suicide, euthanasia and infanticide
Late Christians	Church later altered to the more sophisticated version that the intentional killing of innocent humans was always wrong, whereas it accepted killing in just wars and the lawful execution of criminals, in order to be politically expedient (Rachels, 1986)
Fourth century	In the fourth century further refinement by Augustine proposed that moral goodness was not about the property of actions but was about the attitude with which they are performed: the doctrine of double effect, which will be returned to later (Rachels, 1986)
Seventeenth and eighteenth centuries	In the seventeenth and eighteenth centuries, moral philosophers moved away from religious foundations of morality and proposed that moral truths are known through reason and in the nineteenth century, utilitarians were the first to provide a principled defence of euthanasia (Rachels, 1986)

acceptable, a position also supported by a more contemporary utilitarian, Peter Singer (Singer, 1994). Singer suggests that new commandments should replace certain old ones, and that there should be an acceptance that not all lives are of equal value, that individuals should have the right to decide whether they live or die, and that we should all be responsible for the consequences of decisions that are made regarding end-of-life decisions (Singer, 1994).

Rachels (1986) draws the distinction of having a life (a biographical life) and being alive (a biological life) and considers that if the biographical life is not a worthwhile one then the justification for euthanasia would be apparent – which is where a person is intentionally killed for their own benefit. Hope et al. (2003) further define euthanasia in the following ways:

- **Voluntary active euthanasia**: an action resulting in a person's death which they have completely requested.
- **Voluntary passive euthanasia**: a person is allowed to die (for example, by withholding or withdrawing treatment) which they have completely requested.
- **Non-voluntary euthanasia**: euthanasia when a person is not competent to make a preference known.

This is echoed by Downie & Calman (1994) when they state that in the Judaeo-Christian tradition, the meaning of sanctity of life centres around the person rather than the body and that the Scriptures would not support the maintaining of a body on a ventilator in the absence of a meaningful life. Singer, Rachels and others question the religious premise of the sanctity of life particularly in relation to the clinical needs and effective care of terminally ill patients and in its objections to euthanasia. In the clinical setting the practical application of end-of-life ethical decision making may include the use of:

- Do not resuscitate orders (Figure 7.1)
- Advance directives (Figure 7.2)

It is suggested by Baxter et al. (2002) that 'do not resuscitate' orders are a form of an advanced decision, as the wishes of the patient should be taken into account for a do not resuscitate order to be ethically sound. The only difference is that an advanced decision has been written by the patient in advance of the decision needing to be made, which often allows family members to be more involved as the decision is usually made during less emotional times. When the patient is not competent to

Do Not Attempt Resuscitation (DNAR)

A DNAR decision applies only to Cardiopulmonary Resuscitation. The Chief Medical Officer made it clear (PL/CMO (91) 22) that responsibility for decisions about resuscitation status lies with the consultant in charge of the patient's care, and s/he must consult with the multidisciplinary team. The views of the patients, with due regard to patient confidentiality and the carers should also be considered. In the consultant's absence, a deputy, i.e. Specialist Registrar, may initiate the order providing the consultant is notified as soon as possible.

It is in my clinical judgement that cardiopulmonary resuscitation would not be appropriate for the above named patient for the following reasons:

1. The patient's condition indicates that CPR is unlikely to restore cardiopulmonary function YES/NO

2. CPR is not in accordance with the recorded sustained wishes if a mentally competent patient YES/NO

3. Successful CPR may restore cardiopulmonary function, but is likely to be followed by length and quality of life which would not be acceptable to the patient YES/NO

4. Other (please state)

I have discussed and explained the question of cardiopulmonary resuscitation with the following health care professionals who agree that it would be inappropriate in this case:

(Please complete legibly in BLOCK CAPITALS. Medical staff initiating DNAR should be a Specialist Registrar)

Please note the REVIEW PERIOD overleaf. The frequency of the review period should not exceed one week.

D.N.A.R.
Name of Pt _____
Date _____
Signed _____
This sticker is to be placed in the nursing notes – please refer to medical notes for more details

Figure 7.1   Do not resuscitate orders. Reproduced with permission of Royal Free Hampstead NHS Trust.

Advance Directive
(Personal crisis plan for mental healthcare advance decision making)

You are advised to read the Guidance Notes before completing this document

This is the Advance Directive of: _____ (name)

Address _____

If at any time in the future I experience a mental health crisis, I direct that the following instructions are complied with. In particular, I refuse treatment which is contrary to that stipulated in this document. Where I have objected to a specific form of treatment this shall be legally binding on those treating me, unless I am subject to compulsory treatment under the Mental Health Act 1983.

Signed _____ Dated _____

**Witnessed by ***_____ (name)

of _____ (address of witness)

I confirm that I believe the above named _____ **has freely stated his/ her directions in this document. It is my understanding and belief that s/he has the mental capacity to understand the nature and consequences of these directions.**

Signed _____ Dated _____

*We recommend that you include a witness but this is optional – see Guidance Notes

Issue Number: _____ (If this is the only advance statement you have made enter 1. If this document replaces an earlier version enter 2 and so on)

I have provided a copy of this document to the following people:

_____ (my GP)

_____ (my consultant)

_____ (my partner/spouse)

_____ (family member/s)*
*(If you know who your 'nearest relative' is, include that person here)

_____ (advocate)

_____ (social worker/CPN)

Figure 7.2 Advance directives. Reproduced with permission of
Royal Free Hampstead NHS Trust.

My Wishes regarding medication and treatment:

On previous occasions the following worked well for me:

Things that have not worked well in the past include:

It is my wish that the following people should be told immediately that I have been admitted to hospital:

Other people to contact and tell I am not at home:

I would like the following people to care for my children/dependants until I am able to resume this responsibility myself:

When someone explains my situation to my children I would prefer them to be told the following:

Needs that are special to me which I would like those caring for me to know about: (health/religion/diet etc):

My choice of mental health lawyer* is:
Name/address/telephone number including out of hours contact

*(This should be someone who is qualified to represent you on matters connected with sectioning, compulsory treatment etc. He/she should be a member of the Law Society's Mental Health Panel.)

In the event that I lack capacity to make a decision for myself, I would like the following person(s) to be contacted and consulted:
Name/contact details

I confirm that this person knows and understands the terms of this directive, and that they have given permission to be contacted and will speak for me in a crisis.

Signed

Dated

Figure 7.2 Continued

make a decision then the patient's best interests need to be considered. This often results in the family being involved in the decision, however, the final decision rests with the doctor. In cases where there is no consensus and there is no clear way forward, particularly around withdrawal of treatment, the doctor may seek a judicial review to determine the subsequent medical care.

Prior to the Mental Capacity Act 2005 (Office of Public Sector Information, 2005) there was limited clarity around the legal standing of advanced directives. There was, however, case law (*Re T* (1992)) to support that a person's advance refusal of treatment should be respected. The Mental Capacity Act (2005) which was enforced in 2007 'provides a checklist of factors that decision-makers must work through in deciding what is in a person's best interest'. A person can put his or her wishes and feelings into a written statement if they so wish, which then must be considered. Also, carers and family members gain a right to be consulted. This Act has allowed legal recognition of advanced directives, which in turn reduce the need to seek judicial review when family members are in conflict with the views of the patient. The key principles of the Mental Capacity Act (2005) are as follows:

- People who cannot make decisions for themselves have their rights protected.
- People have their right to be involved and supported in decision making relating to their healthcare protected.
- People can forward plan while able to, by the use of advance decisions ('living wills').
- Nominated others can make decisions on the patient's behalf ('lasting power of attorney').
- Decisions taken by someone else will be in the best interests of the patient.
- A suitable advocate will be provided in the absence of no suitable family or friends.

Slippery slope argument

An important and related concept is the slippery slope argument which raises the fear that permitting voluntary active euthanasia may lead to non-voluntary euthanasia of vulnerable patients, for example, older people or those with learning difficulties (Hope et al., 2003). The slippery slope argument is frequently used in moral discussions about euthanasia as a result of the Nazi atrocities between the 1930s and

1940s (Burleigh, 1995). It is relevant here because for some the distinction between withdrawing life-sustaining treatment and euthanasia is tenuous (English et al., 2004). The logical version of the slippery slope argument is that there would be a logical commitment to extending euthanasia to those who cannot consent and those who may be vulnerable to pressure to consent (Hope et al., 2003). The empirical version asserts that when the constraints on killing are loosened, then undesirable practice will occur (Hope et al., 2003). This last point may be of particular relevance in the removal of non-invasive ventilation from a patient. This may be considered to be 'withdrawal of treatment', however, if killing was more of a norm this could result in unscrupulous decision making based on factors such as age or disability. This may lead to discrimination and may not be in the best interest of the patient and subsequently may occur more frequently and be harder to detect (Kennedy & Grubb, 2000).

Clearly, some believe that we are sliding towards an acceptance of euthanasia (Winterton & Nazarko, 2000), although Griffiths et al. (1998, cited in English et al., 2004) point out that there is no empirical evidence suggesting that rates of non-voluntary euthanasia have increased in the 30 years since euthanasia has been practised openly in the Netherlands. Harris (1985) challenges the slippery slope argument by suggesting that it would be equally immoral if beneficial changes were not implemented because of fear of the presumed dangers.

Doctrine of double effect

The two doctrines of double effect and acts of omissions are often used by healthcare professionals to justify the distinction between voluntary passive and voluntary active euthanasia. The doctrine of double effect was developed in mediaeval Catholic theology and recognised the moral difference between intended and foreseen consequences (Hope et al., 2003). According to the principle it is permissible to produce a bad consequence provided the act in itself is not bad, the bad consequence is not a means to the good consequence and is foreseen but not intended, and there is sufficient reason to allow the bad consequence to occur (Keown, 2002).

The doctrine of double effect provides a defence in end-of-life decisions, where removal of the ventilator may be considered to be a good consequence because its use no longer benefits the patient, but the inevitable and foreseeable outcome (but not the intended one) would be death. Gillon (1985) defends the doctrine because it underlines the fact that to take the utilitarian view that only the consequences of actions are relevant, will fail to account for the conditions in which the action occurred and the intention of the action, which Gillon views as vital to any moral assessment. However, Doyal (1999) points out that intent itself cannot determine the rightness or wrongness of decisions and Harris (1985) also points out that if death is a side effect of treatment that should not diminish the responsibility for it.

Shaw (2002) suggests that the practice of euthanasia is governed more by pragmatic rules than ethics and challenges the relevance of the doctrine of double effect saying that it might be psychologically more comfortable for healthcare professionals to believe that indirect killing has resulted from an action but the flaw in the use of the doctrine is that the person affected by the action is the one who must evaluate its harm and benefit. Finally, both Begley (1998) and Williams (2001) point out that the doctrine has been described as hypocritical and that its validity ethically and legally has been questioned largely because the distinction between intention and foresight is unclear in medical practice, in many instances.

Acts and omissions

The doctrine of acts and omissions claims that failure to perform an act with foreseen bad consequences is morally less bad than performing a different act with identical consequences (Begley, 1998). Deontologists would support the distinction between an act and an omission because in their view what makes an act right is the principle on which it is done while utilitarians would reject such a distinction because of the belief that the outcome must be as good as possible, so it is irrelevant whether this arises from an act or an omission (Singleton & McLaren, 1995). In the example of withdrawing a patient from non-invasive ventilation, it is debatable whether this could be viewed as an act (removal of the patient from the ventilator) or as an omission (omitting to continue to provide burdensome treatment), a dilemma noted by Hope et al. (2003). The doctrines of double effect and acts and omissions define the moral and also the legal distinction (Stauch, 2000) between active and passive euthanasia. However, as both Rachels (1986) and Begley (1998) point out, the moral difference between an act and an omission does not reduce responsibility for the action. In addition, Singleton & McLaren (1995) argue that it is wrong to claim that moral difference is dependent on how the foreseen or intended actions are described.

Case studies

Case study 7.1   Withdrawal of treatment

Bernard is 67 years old and has chronic obstructive pulmonary disease (COPD). He was diagnosed 5 years ago and was recently admitted to his local hospital. He is currently receiving non-invasive ventilation. Initially he used the machine overnight and for short periods during the day to stabilise his arterial blood gases and alleviate his breathlessness. He is now becoming more dependent on it. He enters a stage of total dependence on non-invasive ventilation. The team felt he was now in the terminal stages of his disease and on discussing this with Bernard he did not want to remain on the ventilator.

Ethical considerations: withdrawal of treatment

Decisions relating to the withdrawal of treatment stem mainly from a duty of care to patients to act in their best interests. The three ethical principles of the sanctity of life, the doctrine of double effect and the moral difference between acts and omissions underpin the legal stance to a greater or lesser extent (Hope et al., 2003). There will be times when withdrawal of non-invasive ventilation is considered, especially when the patient is in the terminal stages of their illness. The legal issue that arises is whether the withdrawal of treatment is within the law. In other words is this an active action and therefore active euthanasia or an omission, i.e. passive euthanasia? Montgomery (2003) points out that it is the extent of the duty to act to care for patients, rather than whether euthanasia is active or passive, which must be considered, because if passive euthanasia breaches the duty of care, it is still illegal. However, withdrawal of treatment with consent of the patient as in Bernard's case may be legal provided that the extent of duty of care is fulfilled and is in the best interests of the patient. Numerous authors (Clark, 2002; Hope et al., 2003; English et al., 2004) have suggested that improvements in palliative care would obviate the need for euthanasia and as a result would help to ease the burden placed on patients, family and healthcare teams by poor decision making around end-of-life issues.

Summary

The decision to withdraw the use of non-invasive ventilation is passive euthanasia and as it was in the best interest of Bernard this is legal. The healthcare team were clear that Bernard was terminally ill and they had taken Bernard's wishes into account when making the decision to discontinue the non-invasive ventilation and to keep him on oxygen therapy alone. Palliative care was initiated and the Liverpool Care Pathway was used along with the Gold Standard Framework (Department of Health, 2005) so that community end-of-life support could be instigated in a co-ordinated manner. To withdraw and not to initiate palliative care would not be ethical as this would not be in the best interest of the patient as his symptoms would not have been controlled.

Case law to support decision making (see page 204 for discussion of legal cases):

- The case of Anthony Bland (*Airedale NHS Trust* v. *Bland* (1993)) brought the analysis of acts and omissions into sharp focus and further clarified the position regarding withholding and withdrawing treatment (Kennedy & Grubb, 2000).

Case study 7.2   Advanced decision making

Damian is 24 years of age and has cystic fibrosis. He has always been involved in decision making around the management of his disease and understands how the disease will progress and the impact this will have on him. He has episodes of depression which caused him anxiety as he was very concerned that he would not be able to continue to make decisions about his end-of-life care. In consultation with the healthcare team he decided he did not want to be resuscitated or intubated and that he would like to have his breathlessness controlled with morphine. Damian decided to make an advance directive while he was competent as he was concerned that making his wishes known may become compromised when he was in the terminal stage of his disease.

Damian's condition has deteriorated, resulting in him being admitted to hospital. The healthcare team discusses with the family that Damian is now terminally ill and to control his breathlessness the most appropriate way would be to use morphine. His family become angry and say that they want him to have active treatment, including being resuscitated and being transferred to the intensive care unit as he is so young.

Ethical considerations

- Assessing the competence of patients to make end-of-life decisions.
- Value of advance directives.
- The role of 'do not resuscitate orders' in end-of-life care.

Competence in decision making should involve the following aspects:

- Patients must have the ability to understand the treatment options and be able to express a preference.
- They must be able to cognitively reason how alternative treatments might affect them, remember relevant information and be able to make appropriate decisions.
- Patients should have a concept of what they perceive to be good (for example, they must be able to determine how they value particular outcomes in terms of their benefits or harms).

Hope et al. (2003) suggest that healthcare staff need to assess competence in patients, and that they should therefore follow steps that allow competence in decision making to be established, including:

- Identification of relevant information required by the patient to facilitate their decision making.
- Assessment of the patient's cognitive abilities in term of their understanding, belief in evaluation of the evidence and their consequent ability to make a decision.
- Assessment of other factors which may influence the patient's ability to make a decision (for example, an acute confusional state, mental illness, or lack of cognitive or emotional maturity).

The use of a tool, such as Beauchamp & Childress' (2001) would allow competence within an ethical framework to be assessed (Figure 7.1).

The recognition of **advance decisions** (living wills) by the English and Welsh legal system also challenges the absolute acceptance of the sanctity of life. Advance decisions may be oral, written and may make requests for treatment, or may make a refusal of treatment which is reflected within the Mental Capacity Act (2005).

Do not resuscitate orders are a form of an advanced decision, as the wishes of the patient should be taken into account for a 'do not resuscitate' order if it is to be ethically sound. The only difference is that advanced decisions have been written by the patient in advance of the decision needing to be made, which often allows family members to be more involved as the decision is usually made during less emotional times. There is no ethical or legal duty to seek consent from relatives in 'end-of-life' decision making unless they have been nominated by the patient to act as their advocate. However, their involvement may assist in the overall management of the end-of-life care.

Summary

Although the healthcare professionals were concerned about the expressed wishes of the family, by using ethical decision making they ensured that the decision made was in the best interest of the patient. Through assessing that Damian was competent to make a decision, his wishes were adhered to. The addition of an advanced decision facilitated reaching an appropriate treatment plan that was in the best interest of Damian. If Damian had shared the content of the advanced decision with his family during a less emotional time this may have assisted with the end-of-life discussions. However, this should be Damian's decision, although the healthcare professionals could facilitate such discussions. Even with such preparation the reaction of the family may be the same, as anger is part of the grieving process.

Case law to support decision making (see pages 205, 206 for discussion of legal cases):

- The case of *Re C (Adult refusal of treatment)* (1994) identified that a person with a mental illness could be competent to refuse medical interventions, as it can not be presumed that all people with a mental health problem lack capacity to make decisions.
- The case of *Re T (Adult: refusal of treatment)* (1992) gave a strong indication that a person's advance directive could be binding, dependent on consent or refusal being valid (Kennedy & Grubb, 2000, p. 2034).

Case study 7.3   Voluntary active euthanasia

Harriet is 48 years of age and has motor neurone disease. During a recent chest infection, she was treated with antibiotics. During this acute episode she is commenced on non-invasive ventilation to alleviate her breathlessness. At the time of discharge, a discussion around long-term use of non-invasive ventilation takes place as the healthcare team feels that it may alleviate her distressing symptoms. Harriet states that she did not feel that she was given a choice about starting it, but as she was so ill she did not have the energy to question it. She becomes upset and says that she does not want to be put on the non-invasive ventilator in the future and more to the point feels it is time for her to die. Her husband is with her during these discussions and supports her wishes about her care although is concerned about whether this is possible. On further enquiry about what she meant, she asks for assistance to end her life as she does not want to continue with her life as it is.

Case study 7.3 Continued

Ethical considerations

The ethical principles that need to be considered are:

- Sanctity of life
- Slippery slope argument
- Doctrine of double effect
- Distinction between acts and omissions

Euthanasia can be defined in the following ways (Hope et al., 2003):

- **Voluntary active euthanasia**: an action resulting in a person's death which they have competently requested.
- **Voluntary passive euthanasia**: a person is allowed to die (for example, by withholding or withdrawing treatment) which they have competently requested.
- **Non-voluntary euthanasia**: euthanasia when a person is not competent to make a preference known.

In this case, two forms of euthanasia are being requested.

- Voluntary passive euthanasia (the withdrawal of the non-invasive ventilation) is being requested, which if it is in the best interest of the patient would be legal.
- Voluntary active euthanasia (an illegal act within the United Kingdom and many other countries) as this is asking another individual to assist in the death of the patient.

Summary

Although initially it appeared that Harriet was requesting voluntary passive euthanasia which, given that she was competent to make that decision would be ethically and legally justifiable. However, on further discussion it became clear that she was also requesting voluntary active euthanasia and potentially implicating her husband in an illegal act. This demonstrates the need to explore what patients actually mean when they request that care is ceased.

Case Law to support decision making (see page 203 for discussion of legal cases):

- *R* v. *Cox* (1992) – Dr Cox administered a lethal dose of potassium chloride to his patient with severe rheumatoid arthritis at her request and was found guilty of attempted murder, highlighting the point that in using potassium chloride the doctor had not acted in accordance with proper professional practice (Hope et al., 2003, p. 158).
- *R* v. *Adams* (1957) – Dr Adams was acquitted of murdering an incurably ill, but not terminal patient, by Judge Devlin on the grounds that 'the doctor is entitled to relieve pain and suffering even if the measures he takes may incidentally shorten life' (Mason & McCall Smith, 1999, p. 438).
- *R* v. *Moor* (2000), in which the law supports actions by doctors who believe they have acted properly (Montgomery, 2003, p. 465). Dr Moor was tried and acquitted of giving a dose of morphine likely to contribute to a patient's death (Montgomery, 2003).
- Dianne Pretty *R (on the application of Pretty)* v. *Director of Public Prosecutions* (2002) was one in which the applicant, who had motor neurone disease, wanted the court to allow her husband to help her commit suicide (Baxter et al., 2002, p. 47). The House of Lords and the European Court of Human Rights ruled that this was illegal as it amounted to assisted suicide (Baxter et al., 2002).

Legal cases to support decision making

Standard of care/competent practitioner

Bolam v. *Friern Hospital Management Committee* (1957) established that a doctor must act as a reasonably competent practitioner would have in similar circumstances and that negligence would not be seen to occur if the doctor acted in accordance with a responsible body of medical opinion (Tribe & Korgaonkar, 1993, p. 85). This therefore means that a health professional has a duty to care for a patient where all other reasonable members would do so, but not otherwise (Montgomery, 2003).

Euthanasia

R v. *Cox* (1992), in which Dr Cox administered a lethal dose of potassium chloride to his patient with severe rheumatoid arthritis at her request and was found guilty of attempted murder, highlighted the point that in using potassium chloride the doctor had not acted in accordance with proper professional practice (Hope et al., 2003, p. 158). The judge acknowledged the distinction between intending (potentially murder) and foreseeing (good practice) death by saying that 'the use of drugs to reduce pain and suffering will often be fully justified, notwithstanding that it will, in fact, hasten the moment of death' (Hope et al., 2003, p. 158). He also made the distinction between alleviating distress (even though it might be foreseen that a life might be shortened as a result) and relieving distress through shortening life (Hope et al., 2003).

   R v. *Adams* (1957) illustrated this clearly when Dr Adams was acquitted of murdering an incurably ill, but not terminal patient, by Judge Devlin on the grounds that 'the doctor is entitled to relieve pain and suffering even if the measures he takes may incidentally shorten life' (Mason & McCall Smith, 1999, p. 438). The law clearly condemns active euthanasia as murder because the intent is to kill the patient (Mason & McCall Smith, 1999). In the case of the terminally ill, treatment is directed at the relief of suffering with some risk to life, which introduces the concept of double effect.

   R v. *Moor* (2000) illustrates that the law also supports actions by doctors who believe they have acted properly (Montgomery, 2003, p. 465). Dr Moor was tried and acquitted of giving a dose of morphine likely to contribute to a patient's death (Montgomery, 2003). The judge directed the jury to acquit Dr Moor on the basis that he (the doctor) believed he had given proper treatment to relieve the patient's suffering. Montgomery (2003) points out that the use of a more objective approach, for example, seeking an opinion on professional conduct, may be more appropriate in serious cases such as these.

Withdrawal of treatment

Airedale NHS Trust v. *Bland* (1993) brought the analysis of acts and omissions into sharp focus and further clarified the position regarding withholding and withdrawing treatment (Kennedy & Grubb, 2000, p. 2118). Anthony Bland was a 21-year-old football fan who was injured at Hillsborough football stadium, which resulted in him being rendered permanently unconscious (Montgomery, 2003). After 3 years, the trust applied to the court for a ruling about whether they could discontinue artificial nutrition and hydration, an action which would lead to his death (Montgomery, 2003). The case went to the House of Lords and clarified the point that it may be lawful to withhold or withdraw treatment even if the doctor intends death, if it is in the best interests of the patient to do so and it was argued that withdrawal must be treated as an omission (Montgomery, 2003). This meant that since it was an omission, there was no criminal liability because that would only be the case if there was a duty to act (Montgomery, 2003).

A further point that this case helped to clarify was that there is no legal difference between withholding and withdrawing treatment (British Medical Association, 1999; Luttrell, 1999). The judges in the Bland case acknowledged the illogical distinction between withdrawing life support and killing a patient but considered it a matter for Parliament to reform the law (Kennedy & Grubb, 2000). As a consequence, the House of Lords Select Committee on Medical Ethics was set up in 1994 to consider legal, ethical and social issues at the end of life (Kennedy & Grubb, 2000).

The approach of the courts in making individual assessment of patients' interests may be consolidated by the Human Rights Act 1998 which came into force in October 2002 (Montgomery, 2003), and the courts will now be required to interpret the law consistently with the European Convention of Human Rights (Kennedy & Grubb, 2000). Articles 2 and 3 of the Convention are relevant in the cases of withholding or withdrawing treatment: Article 2 relates to the right to life and Article 3, to the right to protection from inhuman and degrading treatment. Individuals may be able to challenge the withdrawal or withholding of treatment inappropriately if it breaches Article 2 while continuing treatment inappropriately may constitute degrading treatment under Article 3. The impact of these changes cannot be fully assessed yet because the enforcement of the Act is relatively new and the European Court is not bound by precedent as the English courts are (Hope et al., 2003).

Re B (adult: refusal of medical treatment) (2002) established the right of competent adults to refuse treatment and involved a competent patient who wanted life support to be withdrawn and sought the advice of the court which ruled that she had the right to the withdrawal of treatment (Baxter et al., 2002, p. 48).

The case of Dianne Pretty *R (on the application of Pretty)* v. *Director of Public Prosecutions* (2002) was one in which the applicant, who had motor neurone disease, wanted the court to allow her husband to help her commit suicide (Baxter et al., 2002, p. 47). The House of Lords and the European Court of Human Rights ruled that this was illegal as it amounted to assisted suicide (Baxter et al., 2002). On the face of it, as Singer (2002) points out, the two cases share many similarities: both people were competent, rational, and had incurable pathology. The difference between the cases of Ms B and Dianne Pretty rested on the legal right to the withdrawal of treatment even if that means the patient dies and the prohibition of assisted suicide, where no treatment was to be withdrawn, in Dianne Pretty's case.

Re C (a minor) (wardship: medical treatment) (1989) the Court of Appeal approved a course of treatment not aimed at keeping a child alive at all costs (Montgomery, 2003, p. 469).

In *Re J (a minor) (wardship: medical treatment)* (1990) advice was sought from the court about whether a 5-month-old severely brain damaged child should be mechanically ventilated if he collapsed again (Kennedy & Grubb, 2000, p. 2167). Lord Donaldson made the distinction between when a patient is dying whatever the treatment and when the patient is not dying, saying that 'what is in the balance is not life against death, but a marginally longer life of pain against a marginally shorter life free from pain and ending in death with dignity' (Kennedy & Grubb, 2000, p. 2168). Lord Justice Taylor, in trying to determine the quality of the child's life, if treatment was given, talked of whether life would be 'so afflicted as to be intolerable' (Kennedy & Grubb, 2000, p. 2187). Doctors were permitted to allow the child to die.

These two cases (*Re C* and *Re J*) relate to the selective treatment of neonates, underlining the fact that English and Welsh law does not require that life is sustained at all costs whatever the circumstances, rejecting the absolute acceptance of the sanctity of life.

Refusal of treatment

Re T (adult: refusal of treatment) (1992) gave a strong indication that a person's advance directive could be binding, dependent on consent or refusal being valid (Kennedy & Grubb, 2000, p. 2034). Lord Donaldson, in *Re T* confirmed that even if the patient was no longer able to make a competent decision, if the situation had been covered by an advance directive, then a competent refusal of treatment could be binding (Kennedy & Grubb, 2000). Montgomery (2003) points out that the problem with advance directives is that the patient may not be in a position to confirm earlier decisions and again Lord Donaldson stated in *Re T* that where a situation fell outside the scope of an advance directive, then doctors had the 'right and duty' to treat according to what was in the best interests of the patient (Montgomery, 2003, p. 473).

Re C (adult: refusal of treatment) (1994), in which amputation of a leg of a schizophrenic patient was recommended, highlights the need to respect the valid consent or refusal of treatment (Kennedy & Grubb, 2000, p. 2036). The court considered that as the patient could take in, retain, believe and weigh information, balancing the risks and needs, then he was competent to refuse treatment and it accepted the validity of an anticipatory refusal of treatment (Kennedy & Grubb, 2000). Although there is, as yet, no statute law covering advance directives, the Mental Capacity Bill (2004) sets out how they should be applied and, if passed, will enable a lasting power of attorney to be extended to medical decisions and interventions (Dyer, 2004).

Professional responsibility in ethical decision making

The role of rules of professional conduct, such as those developed by the General Medical Council (GMC), the Nursing and Midwifery Council (NMC) and the Chartered Society of Physiotherapy (CSP), will reflect the ethical and legal issues which must be considered in relation to decision making in healthcare (Good Medical Practice (GMC, 2006); Code of Conduct (Nursing and Midwifery Council, 2002); Rules of Professional Conduct of the Chartered Society of Physiotherapy, (CSP, 2002)).

The aims of the rules of professional conduct in relation to ethics are based around the principle-based approach of ethical decision as described by Beauchamp & Childress (2001). These include:

- Assisting healthcare professionals with ethical, moral and legal queries.

- Ensuring patient autonomy is respected (principle of autonomy).
- Guiding healthcare professionals in making ethical decisions that will do no harm and minimising risks to patients (the principles of beneficence and non-maleficence).
- Professional duty of care (the principle of beneficence).
- Treating patients with respect to their rights, dignity and individual sensibilities (rule of fidelity).
- Privileged relationship with the patient (rules of privacy and confidentiality).
- Working in an open and collaborative manner (rule of veracity).

The use of written policies and codes of professional conduct may play little part where decision making must meet the unique requirements of individual situations. Edwards (1996) questions the use of a principle-based approach by saying that its use can be too uncaring and callous with little regard for the moral intuitions and emotions of clinicians. Seedhouse (1998) is also critical of this approach mainly on the grounds that it lacks detail and can therefore be used by anyone to defend anything. Hope et al. (2003) state that we must strive to combine both an intellectual and an emotional response to ethical reasoning.

However, the use of a decision-making framework may assist with making difficult and complex ethical decisions provided that all aspects of a patient's situation are reflected and examined. In relation to patients undergoing respiratory support techniques, there needs to be continuing focus on raising the profile of ethical and legal decision making by improving education and training and enabling opportunities for multi-disciplinary discussions where all those involved in healthcare, including the patients and their carers, feel able to express their concerns and views.

References

Baxter, C., Brennan, M.G. & Coldicott Y. (2002) *The Practical Guide to Medical Ethics and Law*. Pastest, Knutsford.

Beauchamp, T.L. & Childress, J.F. (2001) *Principles of Biomedical Ethics*, 5th edn. Oxford University Press, Oxford.

Begley, A.M. (1998) Acts, omissions, intentions and motives: a philosophical examination of the moral distinction between killing and letting die. *Journal of Advanced Nursing*, **28**, 865–873.

British Medical Association (1999) *Withholding and Withdrawing Life-prolonging Treatment. Guidance for Decision Making*. BMJ Books, London.

Brooks, G. (1997) Advance directives, current legislation and ethical issues. *Nursing in Critical Care*, **2**, 25–28.

Burleigh, M. (1995) *Death and Deliverance: 'Euthanasia' in Germany 1900–1945*. Cambridge University Press, Cambridge.

Chartered Society of Physiotherapy (2002) *Rules of Professional Conduct of the Chartered Society of Physiotherapy*. The Chartered Society of Physiotherapy, London.

Clark, D. (2002) Between hope and acceptance: the medicalisation of dying. *British Medical Journal*, **324**, 905–907.

Dare, T. (1998) Whose life is it anyway? *Nursing in Critical Care*, **3**, 13–16.

Department of Health (2005) Gold Standards Framework (GSF) for Palliative Care. London, HMSO.

Downie, R.S. & Calman, K.C. (1994) *Healthy Respect. Ethics in Health Care*, 2nd edn. Oxford University Press, Oxford.

Doyal, L. (1999) The moral character of clinicians or the best interests of patients? *British Medical Journal*, **318**, 1432–1433.

Dyer, C. (2004) Bill clarifies gap in law over living wills. *British Medical Journal*, **328**, 1516–1517.

Edwards, S.D. (1996) *Nursing Ethics. A Principle-based Approach*. MacMillan, London.

English, V., Romano-Critchley, G., Sheather, J. & Sommerville, A. (2004) *Medical Ethics Today*, 2nd edn. The British Medical Association's handbook of ethics and law. BMJ Publishing Group, London.

Fraser, S.I. & Walters, J.W. (2000) Death – whose decision? Euthanasia and the terminally ill. *Journal of Medical Ethics*, **26**, 21–25.

General Medical Council (2006) *Good Medical Practice*. GMC, London.

Gillon, R. (1985) *Philosophical Medical Ethics*. John Wiley & Sons, Chichester.

Gillon, R. (2003) Ethics needs principles – four can encompass the rest – and respect for autonomy should be 'first among equals'. *Journal of Medical Ethics*, **29**, 307–312.

Harris, J. (1985) *The Value of Life. An Introduction to Ethics*. Routledge & Kegan Paul, London.

Hope, T., Savulescu, J. & Hendrick, J. (2003) *Medical Ethics and Law. The Core Curriculum*. Churchill Livingstone, Edinburgh.

Human Rights Act 1998 [1998] (c. 42).

Kennedy, I. & Grubb, A. (2000) *Medical Law*, 3rd ed. Butterworths, London.

Keown, J. (2002) *Euthanasia, Ethics and Public Policy. An Argument Against Legalisation*. Cambridge University Press, Cambridge.

Lazar, N.M., Greiner, G.G., Robertson, G. & Singer, P.A. (1996) Bioethics for clinicians: 5. Substitute decision-making. *Canadian Medical Association Journal*, **155**, 1435–1437.

Liesker, J., Postma, D.S., Beukema, R.J., ten Hacken, N.H.T., van der Molen, T., Riemersma, R.A., van Zomeren, E.H. & Kerstjens, H.A.M. (2004) Cognitive performance in patients with COPD. *Respiratory Medicine*, **98**, 351–356.

Lloyd, A. (1989) Ethics in intensive care. *Intensive Therapy and Clinical Monitoring*, **10**, 170–175.

Luttrell, S. (1999) Withdrawing or withholding life prolonging treatment. *British Medical Journal*, **318**, 1709–1710.

Nursing and Midwifery Council (2002) Code of Professional Conduct. Available at: http://www.nmc-uk.org

Mason, J.K. & McCall Smith, R.A. (1999) *Law and Medical Ethics*, 5th edn. Butterworths, London.

Montgomery, J. (2003) *Health Care Law*, 2nd edn. Oxford University Press, Oxford.

Office of Public Sector Information (2005) Mental Capacity Act. Available at: www.opsi.gov.uk/acts/acts2005/20050009.htm (accessed 17 May 2008).

Rachels, J. (1986) The end of life. Euthanasia and mortality. Oxford University Press, Oxford.

Ryan, A. (1987) *John Stuart Mill and Jeremy Bentham. Utilitarianism and Other Essays*. Penguin Books, London.

Seedhouse, D. (1998) *Ethics. The Heart of Healthcare*, 2nd edn. John Wiley & Sons, Chichester.

Shaw, A.B. (2002) Two challenges to the double effect doctrine: euthanasia and abortion. *Journal of Medical Ethics*, **28**, 102–104.

Skene, L. & Parker, M. (2002) The role of the church in developing the law. *Journal of Medical Ethics*, **28**, 215–218.

Singer, P. (1994) *Rethinking Life and Death. The Collapse of our Traditional Ethics*. Oxford University Press, Oxford.

Singer, P. (2002) Ms B and Dianne Pretty: a commentary. *Journal of Medical Ethics*, **28**, 234–235.

Singleton, J. & McLaren, S. (1995) *Ethical Foundations of Health Care. Responsibilities in Decision Making*. Mosby, London.

Stauch, M. (2000) Authorship and the equality principle: a defence of acts/omissions distinction in euthanasia. *Journal of Medical Ethics*, **26**, 237–241.

Tribe, D. & Korgaonkar, G. (1993) Withdrawing medical treatment: implications of the Bland case. *British Journal of Nursing*, **2**, 84–86.

Williams, G. (2001) The principle of double effect and terminal sedation. *Medical Law Review*, **9**, 41–53.

Winterton, A. & Nazarko, L. (2000) Debate. Are we sliding towards an acceptance of euthanasia? *Nursing Times*, **96**, 18.

Legal references

Airedale NHS Trust *v.* Bland [1993] 1 All ER 821; [1993] 12 BMLR 64 (HL).

Bolam *v.* Friern Hospital Management Committee [1957] 1 WLR 582.

R (on the application of Pretty) *v.* Director of Public Prosecutions [2002] FLR 268.

R *v.* Adams [1957] Crim LR 365.

R *v.* Cox [1992] 12 BMLR 38.

R *v.* Moor [2000] Crim. LR 31.

Re B (adult: refusal of medical treatment) [2002] 2 All ER 449.

Re C (a minor) (wardship: medical treatment) [1989] 2 All ER 782.

Re C (adult: refusal of treatment) [1994] 1 All ER 819 (Fam Div).

Re J (a minor) (wardship: medical treatment) [1990] 3 All ER 930; [1991] Fam 33 (CA).

Re T (adult: refusal of treatment) [1992] 4 All ER 649; [1992] 9 BMLR 46 (CA).

INDEX

Page numbers in *italics* refer to figures or boxes; those in **bold** to tables